Praise for
The Vintage Remedies Guide to Real Food

"What you eat affects how you feel. It makes perfect sense, yet why is it so hard to find healthy food? Every time you go to the supermarket with your kids, it's a battle, you vs. all of the influences that your children are subject to from the industrial food complex, and I feel like I am losing the war. Along comes natural wellness professional, Jessie Hawkins to the rescue with her second book, writing it as if the reader is having a conversation with her in clear and empowering language.

Ms. Hawkins provides an historical perspective to how we got in this predicament and provides fuel and tools for us to climb out of it, take control, and take better care of our families and ourselves. This is an invaluable aid for all families concerned about health. Jessie reminds us how easy it is to lose sight of the simple fact that health begins with what we put in our body, and, she tells us, very simply, what we should we eat and why we should eat it. This is an amazing tool to have in my Family Medicine practice and to share with my patients. It should be in everyone's shopping cart."

Daniel B. Kalb, MD, MPH, FAAFP
Cool Springs Family Medicine

"I have always believed that feeding each other is one of the most intimate acts we as human beings share with one another. Whether it's a newborn at their mother's breast, a family sharing their evening meal or a potential client offering to buy you lunch to discuss a business deal - they all acknowledge the same fundamental truth – we need nourishment to survive – come let me feed you.

Yet something that is so basic has in recent years - particularly since the early 1970's – become so difficult. In this day of mega grocery marts loaded with every conceivable type of food imaginable – and some that were unimaginable not so long ago – one would be led to believe that good nourishment and thus good health were but a quick trip to the store away. But sadly this is not the case. Where once we had seasonal driven produce we now enjoy virtually anything we want year round – fresh tomatoes at Christmas for example??? And poultry – how do you get a chicken from egg to table in 42 days that weighs 4.5 lbs? Beef – 45% or more increased yield per cow in the last 30 years? Mother nature and good animal husbandry can only do so much – so what accounts for the rest? Genetically modified organisms (GMOs), once the stuff of science fiction, are now the norm. Growth hormones, insect resistant seeds – and on we go. This doesn't take into account the increasingly conflicting information we're bombarded with on a daily basis – good cholesterol / bad cholesterol, good fat / bad fat, good salt / bad salt, etc.

I have tried to live my life in the kitchen – whether cooking for my family, in a restaurant or teaching, adhering to my Grandmother's prime directive – "Son there's better places to save money than the food you put in your family's belly." If you want beef buy real beef. If you want a tomato buy it when God intended it to grow. And my own personal credo – if it says good for you it's probably not, if it says engineered for better health avoid it all costs, and if they have to explain to you why it's not bad for you it most certainly is.

The topics that Jessie address in this book are things that everyone needs to know – not should know – needs to know. I applaud her; I encourage her – read this book.

Chef Jamie Watson
Chef/co-owner, Jamie K's Classique Culinary
Chef Instructor Viking Cooking School, Franklin Tennessee

The Vintage Remedies Guide to:

REAL FOOD

Jessie Hawkins

THE VINTAGE REMEDIES GUIDE TO REAL FOOD
PUBLISHED BY THISTLE PUBLICATIONS
Franklin, Tennessee
a division of Vintage Remedies
www.VintageRemedies.com

ISBN 10: 0-9822318-7-3
ISBN 13: 978-0-9822318-7-6

Warning / Disclaimer: This book is intended as a reference volume only, not a medical manual. Every effort has been made to ensure that the information contained herein is complete and accurate. However, you should consult a physician, preferably a physician with experience in natural medicine before altering your diet significantly, particularly if you have preexisting health concerns. Jessie Hawkins and Thistle Publications / Vintage Remedies shall have neither liability nor responsibility to any person or entity regarding any alleged loss, damage or injury as a result of the information presented in this work. If you suspect that you have a medical problem, please do not delay seeking competent help.

Library of Congress Cataloging-in-Publication Data

Hawkins, Jessie
The Vintage Remedies Guide to Real Food / by Jessie Hawkins
-- 1st Edition
2010922168

ISBN 10: 0-9822318-7-3

Printed in the United States of America
2010, 2012

To my grandmother, Ruth.

My first exposures to real food occurred during my childhood every time I visited my grandmother's house. My grandmother spent her childhood on a farm where her large family grew much of their own food. Knowing the superior flavor of fresh, local foods, she continued her habits long after conventional, processed foods became readily available. While the nation changed to pre-packaged foods and instant shortcuts, my grandmother continued to make her food the "old fashioned" way, confident that it not only tasted better, but was also healthier.

During our visits, I would watch as local farmers brought over bushels of fresh produce throughout the summer. My grandparents were friends with the people that grew their food, and knew their farming methods well. She also kept her own large, varied garden, which kept us little ones occupied during long summer afternoons. With my grandparent's help, I shucked corn, shelled peas, shelled pecans and kept the strawberries safe from invaders, naturally. I learned where my food came from, and how much work was involved in bringing it to my plate.

My grandmother's cooking skills are legendary. She still takes these fresh, basic ingredients and turns them into magical, yet simple meals that nourish all of us. Through her patient lessons with me over the years, I am proud to say I am now following in her footsteps, providing my family with the very best I can serve them.

Thank you GiGi for your loving dedication to your family, and the legacy you continue to provide for all of us to follow.

Contents

ACKNOWLEDGMENTS

I love the way writers are depicted in movies. They sneak off to their secret writing corners, tucked away in a beach house or cabin in the mountains where they allow their thoughts to pour out onto the page, completing entire books in mere weeks. It is always such a dreamy environment, secluded and cozy and, I'm sure, a great atmosphere for writing. Like most careers, however, the depictions are nothing like reality!

My books are completed late at night, when my four children are tucked into bed and I really should be sleeping! They are outlined during homeschooling breaks or tutorial sessions, and they are completed in months, if not years! Yet, despite being a working mommy and wife, these books reflect the collaborative work of many. This book would never be in your hands today without the continued encouragement, feedback and contributions of so many individuals.

Through the endless months I've worked on this project, my husband has helped, pitching in much more than his fair share, with the house, children and even my business. It is only because of his continued encouragement and feedback that this book exists. Thank you Matthew for going above and beyond; I love you.

My children, Gracie, Joel, Micah and Julia also provide feedback as taste testers and "topic creators" as my daily task of caring for them perpetually keeps me on my toes. It is my privilege to be your mother and the lessons you teach me are priceless. Your mommy loves you so much!

My staff at Vintage Remedies continues to wholeheartedly support my goals for the business, ensuring that it consistently thrives smoothly, even in my absence. You guys are amazing and so valuable to me! Thank you Tia Coffey for handling even the most mundane or crazy task with great attention to detail, and Elizabeth Dunne for managing the academic progress of our wellness students. Thank you to Jamey Bennett for once again working your way through my many typos and obscure sentences. Any errors that may remain in this work are entirely my own.

And, of course, this book would not exist if not for the abundant, amazing and awe-inspiring plants and foods placed here lovingly by our Creator. While we continue to learn more about the benefits from our foods, we barely scratch the surface of the complexity of these wondrous gifts He provided for our benefit.

Introduction

My journey into the world of natural health does not resemble the picturesque country life some are blessed to experience. While I definitely had my encounters with real, fresh food, my daily fare was quite conventional. We took full advantage of modern foods, and I had plenty of fast foods during my younger days. My high school years were filled with cola, flavored chips, frozen pizza bagels and baked potatoes with margarine and artificial bacon bits!

Yet, despite my initial habits, becoming a mother encouraged me to reconsider everything I thought I knew about health - and food. I have been on both sides of the fence, fully remembering how it felt to taste organic milk for the first time (I didn't like it!), and making the transition to a healthy, real foods diet. I am personally familiar with the confusion at the grocery store, the struggle to change my palate and the concern about what I am passing along to my little ones.

The benefits from these changes are obvious in my improved health and the health of my family. I have learned to love experimenting with new, fresh ingredients and my taste preferences have (finally) matured as well. I now appreciate the foods I was "forced" to eat as a child, and have now even learned how to make them enjoyable.

If I can do it, so can you! I encourage you to read through this book and work on the traditions you pass along to your children. If your household consumes a conventional diet, these changes may take time. Don't get overwhelmed! Pick your favorite - or what is most important to you - and begin there. Section Three covers how to make this change step by step.

If you already consume healthy, local foods - good for you! You can explore this book, looking for new recipes and techniques for expanding your culinary skills and widen your family's mealtime options.

I am thrilled to see so many families returning to real, healthy foods. This lifestyle has so many benefits that extend beyond our own health and I am thrilled to have you along as I explore each of them!

Section One:
Why we eat...
(...the things we eat)

Chapter One: Food Throughout History

There are few things our bodies truly require on a regular basis for survival. While we may be able to live without air conditioning, soft bedding or even modern houses, none of us would last long without food. A constant supply of nourishing food is one of our most basic needs, and the various methods of providing this need have been a source of much interest, research and study since the beginning of time.

Ancient texts are filled with medicinal and culinary uses for various foods. While religious and cultural influences played important roles in the selection of appropriate foods, they were often matched by the goal of achieving health and wellness. In ancient Egypt, where some of the oldest medical manuscripts have been discovered, the ideas of food, herbs and medicine were nearly indistinguishable. Food was consumed as daily sustenance, but the type of food was only important for medical matters, which included prevention and treatment.

Well-known physicians often promoted their own dietary beliefs. In Egypt, Queen Isis was said to be the keeper of health and gave instruction in the many beneficial plants native to the area. In particular, she promoted the growth and consumption of wheat and barley, as well as fine wines and drinks. Egyptian burial remains also reveal their nutritional beliefs, and the close link between dietary intake and medical health. Many of their medical texts also feature plants for consumption as well as herbs or botanicals for medicinal purposes.

Later, in the prominent Roman Empire, these beliefs were still in place. Emperor Marcus Aurelius' personal physician, the Greek Galen, had some inaccurate theories regarding the digestive process, typically blamed on restrictions on human dissections, but this did not hinder his understanding of the importance of diet and digestive health. He promoted the idea that every food consumed triggers a response within the body, which influenced overall health. His ideas of food affecting health originated in the concept of humors, which was the predominant medical belief of the day, but his ideas about food reflected the minds of many physicians whose names failed to make the history books.

Even Hippocrates, the Greek physician better known as the Western father of medicine, strongly promoted the link between diet and health. His famed saying, "Let thy food be thy medicine, and thy medicine thy food," is still repeated by professionals today. He promoted the use of entire foods as well as herbs for medicinal purposes, and his work strongly influenced countless physicians after his time, including Galen.

These beliefs continued through the discovery of the New World and the study of food and nutrition changed very little between the days of the Egyptian pharaohs, the Greek physicians and early American settlers. Medicines were extracted from herbal plants and certain other foods, and daily food was determined by taste, culture or financial means when illness was not a concern.

For those concerned with the advice of the experts, foods were selected based upon weight and nourishing properties. Without pyramids being taught in grade school health classes, or commercials or public service announcements from special interest groups, the task of choosing the dinner menu was far less complex than it is today. If it was palatable and in style, it would do.

Foods were believed to be whole, inseparable masses of substance. They were judged or evaluated based upon their actions as whole, not individual chemical constituents, which had yet to be discovered. The concept of healthy eating was definitely a well-established field of study, but it looked nothing like our scientific field of nutrition today.

Foods served as fuel, and it was well understood that we needed food on a regular basis. Popular magazines even advised their own ideal intake proportions. One suggested that a woman should consume approximately 20 ounces per day, while a body builder would need roughly 36 ounces. Ounces of *what* were not specified. So, nothing but bread for breakfast and eggs for dinner would do, if the total were roughly 20 ounces.

A New Discovery

Towards the middle of the 19th century, this view of diet that had prevailed for millennia was nearing its demise in many European countries, a change that did not occur in America until several decades later. Once it did, however, it occurred fast, with no looking back. Like never before, experts began to emerge promoting dramatic dietary measures, some beneficial while others were harmful. Magazines began offering health advice based upon some of the popular dietary trends, just as they do today. Apples were a very common remedy as some Americans were consuming meat three times per day with little to no vegetable accompaniment. Of course, this led to digestive complaints, in particular constipation, thus the promotion of an apple as a common remedy was not only popular, but also effective.

What prompted this new group of experts with more dietary advice than experience? A German chemist by the name of Justus von Leibig took some of his dietary theories to the laboratory in the middle 1800s. He felt the body operated much like a machine, and felt there was much more to be understood regarding its fuel. Much of his research revolved around food and agriculture, where he made amazing discoveries. One of which, the calorie, forever changed the concept of whole foods.

Fats, carbohydrates and proteins were also important components of food, and with these discoveries food began its transition from a whole, nourishing mass to an individual group of chemicals. Instead of looking at oranges, tomatoes or peppers, the world began to see water and carbohydrates. Instead of choosing diet by weight or type of food, the notion of meeting individual goals for nutrients began to emerge, forever complicating the way food is selected and consumed.

Of course, as I previously mentioned, Americans were not immediately on board with these new scientific areas of research. As with any historical event, there are multiple reasons for any one occurrence, but one of the contributing factors was the wide division in the way food was regarded in America.

American Diets in the 19th Century

America - the land of plenty. From its infancy, America has been known for its abundance at the dinner table. While gourmet French cooking was born out of the need to make scare amounts of food taste wonderful, and both the French and British were known around the world as culinary greats, America was content to focus on quantity over quality. Many historical texts quote Europeans' disgust when visiting the illustrious New World at the eating habits that prevailed.

Mealtime was not regarded as an enjoyable or relaxing occasion, rather a necessity of drudgery. Perhaps because of the abundance at the table, food was not seen as something worth the expenditure of much effort or time for the sumptuous dishes with elaborate presentations such as those so commonly found in France. The commonality of food made meals more of a hurried task, though with such abundance, the tables overflowed with tasteless but plentiful offerings of food. Not only did this lifestyle fail to please the foreign visitors, it left much food to waste in the process.

Interestingly enough, the abundance of food failed to inhibit the want of plump rounded figures that are so desirable among cultures familiar with poverty and famine. In the late 1800s, one could find entire volumes devoted to the various methods for achieving a large figure, including one book entitled, *How to be Plump*. The actress Lillian Russell, whose hourglass figure earned her the title of America's Beauty, was estimated to weigh approximately 200 pounds! The failure to prepare delicious foods in no way inhibited the desire to consume large quantities.

Nutrition Comes to America

Despite the focus on quantity over quality, a handful of American students had made their way to Germany to study the new field of food science. Inevitably, they brought these new concepts back to the States, not only to change the diets of Americans, but also to turn food science into a profit-making field. With their new expertise and equipment, foods were rushed to the laboratory to be examined and judged for their nutritional worth. The results of these evaluations promoted by the new nutritionists were through various means to reach the masses. Their initial advice? Vegetables, which contained only carbohydrates and water, were essentially worthless for anything other than seasoning. Instead, white flour should be liberally consumed -

white, because the bran was also worthless and should be discarded. Even milk could be improved by condensing it, increasing the sugar content, but reducing the vitamin D content, an unknown result for the researchers of the day. Ideal caloric intake for the average American was set at 3,500 per day.

Fortunately, many Americans disregarded this information. As one participant in a food kitchen experiment remarked, "I'd rather eat what I'd rather. I don't want to eat what's good for me." Had the masses adapted these words of wisdom, it can be safely assumed that disastrous results would have followed. The movement serves as a prime example of the dangers of promoting dramatic changes based upon tiny bits of new scientific information. Our discoveries often merely scratch the surface of an issue, and this can never be misunderstood as providing us the whole picture. The scientific field of nutrition, barely a hundred years old, is still in its infancy, but these initial mistakes serve as stark reminders of the importance to strive for accuracy and a whole picture.

More Nutritional Strides

The field of nutrition and its many misconceptions spread like wildfire on both sides of the Atlantic. Everything from philanthropic projects to infant feeding was changed to conform to the new concepts. Most of these proved to be disastrous, but the changes continued nonetheless. For most Americans, the problems with nourishment were completely unrelated to finances, but were entirely related to dietary trends and social conformity.

Nonetheless, the field of nutrition learned from many mistakes and continued to discover nutrients that were both valuable and critical to the human diet.

Eventually, these discoveries expanded to include enzymes, phytonutrients, antioxidants and other beneficial substances that don't necessarily qualify as vitamins or minerals. Yet, despite these advancements, the field still has much room to grow and develop. There are many compounds within whole foods that have yet to be identified and many with benefits yet to be discovered. For these reasons, we can learn from the discoveries of nutrition, while fully understanding the limitations it has, and instead of relying on individual nutrients or supplements for nutrition, focusing on real, whole foods with benefits yet undiscovered.

Chapter Two: Nutritional Basics

Despite the field of nutrition being relatively new, much of the information that has been uncovered can be useful and applicable when examining dietary habits and food. In this chapter, the basics of nutrition will be covered. While many of these principles and guidelines are quite valid, there is some ground that is still new or unclear. In those circumstances, my general rule of thumb is to stick with what is traditional and natural. By traditional, I'm not referring to the food we consumed as children. I'm talking about the preparations methods and consumption habits that were shared by countless generations before us.

The understanding of the chemical composition and biological effects of our food supply serves to enhance the understanding of dietary health, not to change the habits that sustained previous generations for millennia.

Proper nutrition can help keep the body healthy, ensuring that it not only has the ability to fight off infection and illness, but that it can grow and age appropriately. Yet, so few individuals actually learn real nutrition in school or in life. Special interest groups present most nutritional informational available to the public. We have been given pyramids, squares and other assorted shapes, but none of these actually define healthy eating, and they leave more room for confusion than explanation. When this is combined with virtually unregulated advertisements coming from every direction, in an environment where it is better to ask forgiveness than permission, and even school lunches provided for children that don't meet even the most basic nutritional standards, true nutrition is elusive at best.

Yet, nothing could be simpler. The confusion is only a result of attempts to combine science with financial interests, and the gross over-complication of essential concepts. In the classes I teach, the most important nutritional concept we present is the idea of holistic nutrition. This means that there is no "one size fits all" answer to nutritional guidelines. Some individuals have physical needs, such as a pregnancy, that will dictate the guidelines to a healthy diet; others have personal preferences or religious beliefs that set the standard for food. And our bodies, being uniquely fearfully and wonderfully made, were not designed to always eat what our neighbor eats. However, there are certain aspects that are applicable to everyone. Each of us needs protein, fats and carbohydrates on a daily basis. Each of us needs essential vitamins, minerals, enzymes and assorted phytonutrients.

Real Food Composition

When food is broken down to its individual particles, two main categories emerge: macronutrients and micronutrients. Macronutrients are the compounds that comprise the basic elements of food. These include fats, carbohydrates and proteins. While most individuals have been taught that only one of those three items is desirable and healthy, the truth is that all three are of equal importance. In smaller quantities are the micronutrients. These are the vitamins, minerals and other elements that are crucial to health, but are not consumed in such large amounts. There are even micronutrients that are yet to be discovered, which is another great reason to consume foods fresh and whole, instead of focusing on individual compounds, which has gotten society into trouble in the past.

Carbohydrates

Carbohydrates were considered to be a very important part of a well-rounded diet until the low-carb craze took over. Unfortunately, eliminating or reducing carbohydrate intake for the sole purpose of weight loss is neither healthy nor productive, according to scientific study. While carbohydrate intake may be a real problem among those who consume a conventional diet, a better solution is to change the diet to include healthy and beneficial carbohydrate choices, reducing or (ideally) eliminating the poor quality processed foods, not the entire classification.

Technically, carbohydrates are hydrated chains of carbon. Carbohydrate production is a simple, but amazing, recurring cycle. It begins when plants take carbon dioxide from the air and combine it with water, using the energy provided by the sun. This process is known as photosynthesis, which means "putting together." As this occurs, oxygen is released into the air. When we consume oxygen, we burn it as fuel with carbohydrates, releasing the energy contained within. This produces carbon dioxide and water, which we release, beginning the process again.

In more practical terms, carbohydrates are necessary for human survival. Our bodies require greater amounts of carbohydrates than any other nutrient. Every part of the body requires carbohydrate intake, and the central nervous system and red blood cells use glucose exclusively for optimal functioning. In addition, carbohydrates serve as communication devices in the body. Essentially, sugars help our cells interact with each other. They play a role in immune function and can even affect the formation or prevention of tumors.

Yet, all of these great benefits are only obtained from healthy carbohydrates. Refined, stripped, bleached and processed carbohydrates not only fail to provide these benefits, they adversely affect the body, creating problems with insulin metabolism, weight gain, liver health, cognitive functioning, immune health and daily energy levels. These unhealthy carbohydrates are easily identified, as they can be found in refined flours, processed sugars, most baked goods, anything with "white" in the title, and most desserts or treats. They are also present in so-called healthy snacks such as pretzels, crackers, cheese snacks and other dry baked goods.

One important guideline that I repeat often is that consuming healthy foods should not be based on what *not* to do, but what to do. So, a list of what not to consume may have its place, but a list of good choices is more beneficial and useful. So, no carbohydrate discussion would be complete without looking at some yummy and healthy options for carbohydrate intake.

Of course, fruits and vegetables are always healthy sources of nutrients, including carbohydrates. Anytime I see a diet plan that restricts intake of fresh fruits and vegetables without allergy or sensitivity issues being present, a big red flag goes up. Plant based diets are by far the healthiest diets one can adapt. This does not necessitate a vegetarian diet; it is easily possible to include meats in a plant-based diet, but produce should be an important part of every diet. Other healthy carbohydrates include whole grains, with emphasis on the word *whole*.

These healthy carbohydrates include the nutrients necessary for their digestion and metabolism, unlike the refined versions, which strip the body of nutrients. While refined carbohydrates can affect insulin production and sensitivity adversely, some healthy carbohydrate choices can have the opposite effect, improving blood sugar metabolism.

Additionally, healthy carbohydrates include fiber. This substance, known as roughage, is resistant to human digestion, sweeping the intestines clean. The World Health Organization recommends an absolute minimal daily intake of 25-40 grams of fiber, but most individuals only consume about half of that. Diets rich in plant based foods and healthy carbohydrates can easily obtain twice those numbers, without even trying.

Why is fiber so important? In addition to cleansing the bowels, it helps maintain health. Smooth digestion prevents hemorrhoids and appendicitis. It also reduces cancer rates and prevents many emotional disorders. Fiber can help correct cholesterol ratios, lowering the amount of "bad" cholesterol.

It also helps to ensure healthy intestinal flora, which is the term used to describe the type of microbes that live in the gut and bowels. Humans are individual ecosystems, literally home to billions of microbes, including bacteria. Most bacteria are beneficial to the human body, but a few varieties can be harmful or even cause infection. One great way to prevent colonization by these unfriendly bacteria is to ensure that the friendly bacteria population is thriving. Fiber contributes to the growth and health of the friendly type of bacteria. If the digestive system is sluggish or slow, the rotting waste encourages the growth of the unfriendly bacteria, which have the ability to cause numerous health concerns.

Even with healthy carbohydrate choices, consumption should be balanced by healthy fats and proteins. This is best achieved with a balanced, varied diet, not by counting grams of anything throughout the day. Of course, misinformation has also been spread about both protein and fats, so I'll cover those next.

Fats

Before the low carb craze existed, the low fat craze was strong. These fads don't correct themselves quickly, so many still assume that fats are just as terrible as carbohydrates. Interestingly enough, the low fat craze is probably what led to the low carb craze, as the fats were often replaced with poor quality carbohydrates, leading to the over-indulgence of unhealthy carbohydrates. Yet, just as carbohydrates have been misunderstood, fats are much more valuable than they first appear.

Fats are divided into many classifications, based on their molecular structure. These include saturated and unsaturated, which are then classified as mono- or polyunsaturated, and long chain, medium chain and short chain, which are not as commonly identified on food labels.

A fat becomes saturated when all of its available openings on the chain are taken with hydrogen. If there are open spots, the fat is known as unsaturated. This leaves unsaturated oils vulnerable to rancidity, which occurs when oxygen takes the available spot on the chain, hastening the deterioration process. Distinguishing between saturated and unsaturated fats doesn't require a home laboratory; the saturation increases the melting point of the fat, causing it to become solid at room temperature. So, butter, coconut oil, palm oil, lard and other solid fats are saturated. Olive oil, safflower oil and flax oil are all unsaturated.

When saturated fats first began to earn a bad reputation, an old, cheap butter substitute, known as margarine, suddenly became the "new" health food. This substitute involved taking an unsaturated fat and putting it through a process known as hydrogenation, which artificially saturates the fat. This process was hailed as a nutritional advancement, but the reality is that hydrogenated oils cause quite a bit of harm. This is one of those examples where the natural and traditional way would have been superior to the prevailing theories of the day. Fortunately, the dangers of hydrogenated oils are becoming well known, and many companies are turning back to natural options.

These natural options include both saturated fats and unsaturated fats because both fats are important to human health. The body uses both types of fat in different ways, which are not interchangeable. In other words, if you eliminated one type of fat, the other kind would not be able to perform the same functions. With the exception of the central nervous system and red blood cells, every system in the body requires fat for energy, and over two-thirds of the brain is composed of fat! Children, in particular, need sufficient fat intake for proper cognitive functioning.

So, if the body needs fats on a regular basis, which type of fat should be consumed? Naturally occurring fats are a must - so no hydrogenated or otherwise altered fats. Plant based fats are healthier than animal fats, although the fat from free range, grass fed, hormone and antibiotic free animals would be far superior to conventional animal fat. In fact, mammals tend to store toxins in fatty tissues; so the fat of conventional factory raised animals would be a concentrated source of assorted harmful toxins.

Due to the potential for rancidity, my personal rule is to consume unsaturated fats primarily at room temperature or in preparations that require little heat. This includes vinaigrettes, bread dipping sauces, assorted condiments and some sautéed dishes. For high heat such as frying or any sustained heat, I use a saturated fat such as coconut oil or palm oil. This allows me to enjoy the best properties of each fat and prevents potential rancidity or oxygenation from occurring during the cooking process.

In addition, two oils are essential for the diet. These are known as essential fatty acids or by their names, omega 3 and omega 6. These two oils perform important functions within the body, one (omega 6) contributing to the natural inflammatory response, while the other (omega 3) has anti-inflammatory effects. Unfortunately, most individuals consuming a conventional diet are obtaining more than enough omega 6 oils, but not enough omega 3 oils. The two should be consumed in a balance to maintain the inflammatory response.

To correct this, many individuals supplement with fish oils or flax oil. Many health concerns are related to insufficient omega 3 oils. These include high cholesterol, diabetes, heart disease, obesity, arthritis, osteoporosis, depression, bipolar disorder, ADHD, various eating disorders, skin conditions such as eczema, irritable bowel syndrome, macular degeneration, PMS, cancer, asthma, lack of attention and poor energy levels. (You may notice that many of these concerns are related to inflammation.) Balancing these fats plays a critical role in many common, and often overlooked, body functions! Many of the descriptions in the food guide towards the end of this book will provide information on foods that are rich in omega 3 oils.

Protein

Proteins are known as the building blocks of our bodies. Few would question the importance of protein in the diet, as it is crucial for new growth and development, particularly among pregnant women and children. However, most individuals don't realize that protein is readily available in both plant and animal foods.

A protein is a long strand of one hundred or more amino acids. Our bodies do not produce some of these amino acids, thus they are essential to the diet. With little exception, animal foods are the only sources that provide all of the essential proteins in one place, preventing deficiencies from occurring. However, plants contain an array of amino acids, and as long as the diet is varied, vegetarians have no trouble obtaining sufficient protein and essential amino acids from plant sources. Some plant sources, such as quinoa, even contain all of the essential amino acids in one place, but this is typically rare. To compensate for this, many professionals previously recommended food combining, which blended foods with different amino acid profiles together in the same meal so that the body could receive all of the essential amino acids in a single meal, but further research has shown that the body knows how to handle them as they come and it is not necessary for anyone to worry about combining foods at each meal. However, it is important to ensure that the diet is varied to prevent deficiencies.

Due to the poor reputations of fats and carbohydrates, proteins have received a bit more than their fair share of attention. Very few individuals actually have deficiencies in protein, but the over-consumption of protein is not uncommon. Nutritional guidelines for protein consumption vary, but are consistently on a downward trend. Research has shown that pregnant women and growing children need to focus on protein consumption, but everyone else would probably benefit from consuming *less* protein.

This requires an approach to meals that is not focused on the traditional "meat and two sides." Instead, most individuals would benefit from consuming meat two to four times a week, resembling the diets consumed by many of our ancestors, when meat was expensive and scarce. Adjusting the meat intake to a proper place in the diet also makes room in the budget for better quality meat.

The days without meat would not be void of protein. On the contrary, most individuals receive ample amounts of protein from plant sources without even realizing it. Using a hamburger as an example, not only does the meat provide protein, but also the bun, tomato, lettuce and even some condiments are contributing to the total protein count of the meal. Focusing on plant-based proteins will also typically result in an increase of fiber intake, which brings about numerous additional health benefits.

Great protein sources include grains, nuts, beans, legumes, free range, grass fed, antibiotic and hormone free meats, fish and even many vegetables. Poor quality animal products, if used as the primary source of protein in the diet, can adversely affect health in many ways. Simple changes to the type and quality of meat and the abundance of plant-based proteins can bring about amazing health benefits.

Vitamins

Vitamins are perhaps the most well known of the micronutrients. These are extremely new to the fiend of nutrition, and were named for their importance, literally meaning "vital for life." To become classified as a vitamin, the substance must be found to be essential for survival. If the substance is not found in the diet, adverse health events follow. These are not as common today, as most modern deficiencies are mild, not severe, but when nutrition was new, and fruits and vegetables were not considered to be important, problems such as beriberi and rickets were not as far removed.

Many individuals study vitamins and minerals, then immediately feel the need to go purchase high potency supplementation to receive these benefits, but this approach is not advised and could even be harmful. Multivitamin supplements are useful, especially considering the nutrient depletion of most conventional crops. (Studies have revealed that organic produce is far more nutrient rich than conventional counterparts.) But, vitamin and mineral intake is a careful balancing act. Many vitamins are lipid soluble, which means that an overdose is possible. Likewise, many minerals need to be taken in balance with another mineral, as the two share receptor sites, and increased intake of one can lead to deficiencies of another. Additionally, the mega dosage of vitamins or minerals is no longer under the classification of supplementation; it is using the substance as a medicinal drug, which should not be undertaken without the assistance of a competent care provider, preferably someone trained in holistic health.

Each vitamin and mineral has an RDA, which is often set as the ideal goal, but this topic is seen differently among natural health professionals. The standards were set to reflect intake that prevents deficiency, not as a goal for optimal health. It was never meant to be the ideal intake for maximum health, nor was it set to be a maximum intake as it is often considered. It merely helps to prevent deficiencies that may cause severe health consequences. Yet, so few individuals meet even these minimums.

Like the macronutrients, spending the day counting and measuring intake is not the best way to obtain a healthy diet. Instead of focusing in the numbers, the focus should be on the variety and quality of the diet.

The most common vitamins are vitamin A, B complex, C, D, E and K. Vitamin A, also known as retinol, is a fat-soluble nutrient that is known for benefiting the health of the eyes. It is said to help alleviate night blindness. It also helps boost the immune system, and studies have found that children with low levels of vitamin A are more prone to intestinal and respiratory infections.

The B complex family of vitamins includes several different nutrients, all of which benefit emotional health and cognitive functioning, when sufficient amounts are included in the diet. Unfortunately, low levels of B complex vitamins are quite common. The refining and processing of many foods remove the B vitamins, so making a change to whole grains and real foods will help prevent this.

These low levels have been linked with increased risk of anemia, and diabetics, alcoholics and children with special needs all have a need for increased intake of B complex vitamins. Vitamins in this family include thiamin (B1), riboflavin (B2), niacin (B3), pantothenic acid (B5) pyridoxine (B6), folate (B9) and cyanocobalamin (B12).

Ascorbic acid is another water-soluble vitamin, better known as vitamin C. This nutrient is important to many body functions and has become fairly well known recently because of its impact on the immune system. It also helps with collagen production and speeds the recovery time for those with poorly healing wounds. It plays a role in alleviating allergies, bacterial and viral infections.

Another vitamin that helps prevent colds and infections is the fat-soluble vitamin D, also known as the sunshine vitamin. Recent research shows that many individuals have extremely low levels of vitamin D, which some attribute to the overuse of sunblock, preventing the absorption of vitamin D. While sunblock is helpful for skin cancer prevention, moderate sun exposure can also be healthy. In addition to the increased susceptibility to colds, low levels of vitamin D adversely affect bone health.

Vitamin E, also known as alpha tocopherol, is a somewhat controversial vitamin as some argue that it is not absolutely vital to life. However, it plays an important role in fertility, the prevention of heart disease, maintenance of healthy skin and detoxification. As an antioxidant, it is also beneficial when added to oils that are prone to rancidity as it can lengthen the shelf life of such oils. While vitamin E is lipid soluble, it does not appear to build up in the body as other lipid soluble vitamins.

Minerals

While daily intake of minerals is quite scarce, these little substances have many beneficial actions in the body, despite their small size. Even trace minerals like zinc have been shown to play important roles in the body - without it, the entire process of eliminating CO2 would be dysfunctional.

Minerals also interact with each other, and the surplus or deficiency of one can affect many other minerals. Whole, real foods tend to supply these minerals in the healthy ratios our bodies require, and are also the most bioavailable sources of minerals.

The most abundant mineral in the body is **calcium**, which is vital to bone health, but is constantly being leached from the body. Calcium absorption is both helped and hindered by protein, and vegetarians often have better bone health than omnivores because of this. Calcium is often available with a **magnesium** supplement, so the two can be found in a healthy balance. Unprocessed, real foods such as whole grains are great sources of magnesium and shortages are not uncommon. Refined grains are often extremely lacking in magnesium.

Sodium and **potassium** also have a balancing act as they help to regulate bodily fluids. They are known as electrolytes and are often found in drinks marketed towards athletes. The modern processed diet adversely affects this ratio as it provides more sodium without sufficient potassium.

Another mineral pair, **zinc** and **copper**, are often found in unbalanced ratios. Due in part to the abundance of copper pipes for the water supply, many individuals had zinc deficiencies, which can lead to decreased appetite, skin conditions and developmental delays, but not everyone needs zinc supplementation.

Other important minerals include phosphorus, manganese, chromium and iron. Most modern diets are deficient in many of these important minerals, particularly iron, which is important to healthy energy levels, childhood development and even immune health, and chromium, which helps regulate blood sugar levels and helps digest sugars.

In addition to these micronutrients, many other ingredients in food have been discovered since the introduction of nutrition. These include enzymes, which help with digestion, antioxidants, which are important for detoxification and cancer prevention, and phytonutrients, which are plant based nutrients.

While supplementation with individual nutrients, vitamins or minerals may seem to be the solution to ensuring that everyone has sufficient intake, there is no way to identify individual ideal intake of any nutrient, and everyone benefits from a diet rich in real foods, naturally providing these nutrients in their natural ratios, ready for optimal absorption.

Chapter Three: Why Food Matters

The last chapter covered the benefits of various nutritional compounds within foods. Obviously consuming poor quality foods deprives the body of these great benefits, but the impact of the modern food supply goes deeper than the deprivation of nutrients. These so-called foods not only leave a void, they cause harm and alter the body in such a way that the low levels of nutrients are magnified. Some processed foods can even aggravate the nutritional loss, increasing the daily intake required for optimal health. These factors may not receive the attention they should, but when the importance of a real foods diet is realized, real health can occur. Many clients and students of mine are astonished at the improvements to their health or their family's health that appear after making simple adjustments to the diet.

Most people are under a misconception that poor quality foods may be bad for the waistline, or diagnosed health problems, but aside from those concerns, food is unimportant. Nothing could be further from the truth. Not only is the waistline a poor indicator of health - our country is filled with overweight malnourished individuals - every part of our being depends on nourishment provided by the diet on a daily basis. Depriving the body of essential nutrients can have disastrous consequences, and many processed and refined foods strip the body of nutrient stores, causing further depletion.

The medical reports on television are filled with phrases such as "obesity epidemic" and "increasing rates of..." cancer, diabetes, childhood obesity, autism, celiac, intestinal disorders, depression, infertility, learning delays and many other concerns. What is causing the dramatic increase in these modern epidemics? Why are these numbers steadily increasing, not decreasing? The factors are complex, but the current standard diet plays an important role.

The Standard American Diet (S.A.D.) is filled with hydrogenated oils, high fructose corn syrup, and foods that have been modified and processed at numerous stops between the farm they may have originated on and the dinner table. Each of these stops increases the risk of contamination by both indirect additives and microbial pathogens. Each stop lengthens the distance between the source and the table, which often decreases nutrient content, and each of these stops uses valuable resources that are diminishing. The current food model is unhealthy and it is unsustainable. It cannot continue as it is and - even if it could - we cannot continue consuming these imitation foods.

Not all Fuel is Equal

Everything that is put into the body requires a response. It is not merely digested and discarded, with anything good being absorbed and anything bad merely passing through. Every single thing must be evaluated, processed and digested or metabolized.

Our bodies, as you probably know, are technically hollow. We are like tall doughnuts, and the foods we eat go through the middle of the doughnut. Some things, like fiber, sweep that center clean, preventing build up of waste or toxin forming matter, but other things are absorbed into the actual body and when this occurs, the body must react.

If the food provides the nutrients necessary for its metabolism and assimilation, the body benefits from the use of these nutrients as fuel, building blocks or other important factors in the ongoing process of maintaining homeostasis. If the food, such as a refined sugar, does not provide the necessary tools for its processing, the body must rob from its stores to metabolize the food. When this occurs, deficiencies are created, as the food resulted in an overall loss of nutrients. To maintain healthy bodies, the foods consumed need to be depositing, not withdrawing, nutrient stores within the body.

Other foods may not rob the body of nutrient stores, but prevent the use of healthier options, resulting in less than optimal bodily functioning.

Hydrogenated Oils and Trans Fats

Oils are necessary for optimal cognitive functioning, yet the body has specific requirements for these oils, which are not interchangeable. The brain is composed of approximately 2/3 fatty acids, and fatty acids are the most crucial dietary molecules in the brain. In other words, the brain requires fatty acids for optimal functioning and anything related to cognitive functioning, including age related memory loss, depression, bipolar disease, Alzheimer's disease, childhood development (particularly regarding reading abilities, spelling, auditory memory, speech and overall intelligence) and dementia are all dependent on the availability of these healthy fats.

These healthy fats are the omega oils that have become so popular lately, and it is no secret that most individuals with modern diets lack these nutrients. However, the abundant intake of hydrogenated oils and trans fats is a major contributing factor to this problem.

Trans fats, which are produced in the hydrogenation process, have the ability to cross into the brain. Once there, they adhere to receptor sites for DHA. In other words, they have crashed the party and are taking the seats intended for the healthy brain fats, including DHA. This inhibits the body from realizing the benefits of DHA. Furthermore, studies in rats revealed that when trans fats were combined with low levels of omega 3 fatty acids, the uptake of trans fats into the brain doubled.

This affects the neurotransmitter dopamine, which is associated with pleasure and enjoyment. It also blocks the body's ability to produce its own DHA, a process that naturally decreases with age, so it may be able to hasten the aging process, particularly as it relates to cognitive functioning. It causes unhealthy cholesterol ratios, increasing the "bad" cholesterol and decreasing the "good" cholesterol, and may even affect the brain's blood supply.

Trans fats not only have the ability to cross into the brain, they can also cross through the placenta and enter the developing brain of an unborn child, and they cross through breast milk to the brain of a nursing baby. Many studies have revealed that babies born to mothers with healthy supplies of omega fatty acids have better eyesight and cognitive functioning than control groups.

These concerns have lead many regulators to focus on the abundance of trans fats in the diet, limiting or preventing their use in restaurants. Trans fats offer no nutritional value, only potential risks, so there is no harm in eliminating them from the diet, and the benefits are significant.

High Fructose Corn Syrup

Another common ingredient that even has a natural sounding name is high fructose corn syrup, also known as HFCS. This sugar substitute has become popular among food manufacturers primarily because it is inexpensive. HFCS can be found in products ranging from children's drinks to sodas to pretzels and other so called "healthy" snack foods.

Yet, is HFCS safe? Many questions have been raised lately and many studies seem to conclude otherwise. The concerns with HFCS are focused around two key areas, the fructose content and the quality of the corn, though another potential concern is the presence of trace levels of mercury that were recently found in HFCS.

HFCS is overly processed to contain higher levels of fructose. Fructose is metabolized by the body differently than glucose and has been linked with diabetes, obesity, insulin resistance and related concerns. Fructose increases the desire for more food, whereas glucose sends signals to the body that its current energy needs have been satisfied.

It also is typically made from poor quality GMO corn, with pesticide residue and other indirect additives. Grains accumulate pesticides and other toxins in the kernel, so concentrations of these contaminants as high as ten fold are common, and even one hundred fold are not unheard of.

Pesticides and Organics

While not an intentional ingredient, the use of pesticides and other agricultural compounds in conventional produce play key roles in the overall health of an individual food. While many assume that the benefits of organic revolve around the omission of pesticides and additives, which are certainly great benefits, these are only the starting point.

Organic farming reduces many of the most important food safety concerns, particularly pesticide safety, antibiotic resistance and GMO risks such as allergens. The other two of the five most common risks include bacterial contamination and mycotoxins, and organic farming habits can help, but not alleviate these concerns.

Furthermore, and perhaps most important to families, organic produce is more nutrient dense than conventional counterparts, according reviews of over 100 published studies. In practical terms, this means that consuming a single apple or serving of green beans will provide more nutrients if an organic apple or serving of green beans is chosen over conventional. For every fruit or vegetable our children consume, they will receive more benefits if it is organic than conventional. To flip the tables, it would take more conventionally raised produce to meet the nutritional needs of a growing child than organic produce.

This nutritional superiority includes increased concentrations of vitamins, minerals, antioxidants, polyphenols and fewer nitrates. In some cases, the antioxidant capacity was 88% higher in organic produce! This is a significant difference.

While most studies are from the viewpoint that organic produce offers more nutrients, when food history enters the picture and previous farming methods are evaluated, one could conclude that produce is much less nutrient dense than in previous generations. Over time, due to conventional farming methods combined with poor quality - which is also related to conventional farming methods - the nutritional value of food has decreased.

Organic farming is important to meet current nutritional needs. It also increases soil quality, ensuring that the food system is sustainable and the soil we farm can still provide nutritious foods for our children's children. It increases worker safety for those employed by farmers and it increases the nutritional content of the meals at the table.

Chapter Four: Targeting Children: The Disastrous Results of Modern Food

While diet is important to all of us, there is one group of individuals who are more susceptible to the harmful effects of the various additives, preservatives and synthetic chemicals that are present in our current food supply. Adults may be able to manage limited exposure effectively, but children have unique traits that make them far more susceptible than the rest of us.

For an adult, most of the dietary intake is used to sustain the current body mass and maintain homeostasis. With the exception of pregnant women and body builders, adults have finished growing. Our body systems are mature, and all of our development is complete. Even our mental growth is different, as our days are not typically spent learning and memorizing facts as a grade school student. When we are exposed to toxins or poor quality foods, our bodies have the ability to withstand it for moderate periods of time. Build up to the point of disease may take months or years, but often, exposure can be repaired over time.

Children, however, do not have those abilities. Their rapid rate of growth means that their bodies are taking in more food per pound than an adult would. This is especially evident during the first few months of life, when an infant will double his or her birth weight. No adult is consuming amounts of food intended to double their weight. Even after that time period, children are growing at rapid rates, requiring large intake of food in comparison to their current size.

Of course, consuming more food per pound means that more nutrients are needed for the body to grow and develop properly. If the food lacks nutrients or contains pesticides, additives or potentially harmful toxins, that exposure will be compounded as well. This means that even moderate intake has a larger influence than it would for an adult, whose intake is intended to merely maintain current body mass.

The rate of rapid growth also leads to another potential problem with exposure to poor quality or processed foods and additives. For the body to achieve the growth intended for that window of time, it will need certain nutrients. If those are not available, development is hindered. Furthermore, if exposure to substances that inhibit development occurs during this critical phase, the body has to halt the natural growth phase temporarily to process the exposure, potentially hindering development, even if proper nutrients are available. In some cases, the window for development can pass, and certain milestones or traits may never be reached. For adults who are no longer growing and developing, this issue is not a concern.

Furthermore, the metabolic pathways in children are not fully mature. What this means in practical terms is that they are not able to fully detoxify exposures to synthetic chemicals, pesticides or additives that are often found within processed foods. This inability to excrete the exposures leaves children susceptible to their harmful effects in greater levels than their adult counterparts.

Finally, their young age means that these toxins that are not excreted are able to build up within the body. This longer build up period means that approaching the damage threshold is more of a possibility than an adult with fewer years of exposure in their systems. For example, if a particular exposure takes ten to twenty years for symptoms to appear, an adult may be in his or her forties or fifties before symptoms begin. With childhood exposures, this could occur during a person's twenties or thirties. For substances with shorter build up periods, this would increase childhood diseases. This partially explains the increase of many childhood diseases that were usually limited to the adult population in previous generations. While cancer and other serious illnesses are possibilities, some of the largest increases have been seen in chronic illnesses, with mild but constant symptoms.

Even when processed foods with additives have been eliminated from the diet, children remain vulnerable to poor dietary choices, as their digestive systems are often still quite immature. The ability to process the strong proteins in cow's milk and certain other foods may not exist yet, and the introduction of these foods too early may affect future development. For this reason, many childhood development experts recommend waiting until the child is 12 months old to consume some difficult to digest foods, but many experts advise waiting even longer to prevent the development of sensitivities or allergies, and ensure a healthy digestive process for the child's future.

When these steps are not followed, many children show their difficulty in processing such foods with symptoms like chronic ear infections, eczema and other skin conditions, irritability, fatigue, irregular bowel habits such as diarrhea or constipation, impaired cognitive functioning such as distractibility or inability to concentrate, and numerous other complaints.

Kid Friendly Foods

Given the above information, it would seem that the healthiest foods would be marketed towards children - in an ideal world. Yet, we don't live in an ideal world, and our harsh reality is that the average "kid friendly" options are anything but healthy for optimal growth and development.

Children are reputable picky eaters, but what we often fail to remember is that we have control over what tastes they develop - even at a very young age. Events and venues aimed at serving children typically provide hot dogs, macaroni and cheese, pizza, chips, French fries and soft drinks. If adults are present, a salad bar or salmon entree may be added to the mix for the more mature palate. Even in family friendly restaurants, the child's menu typically features the exact same fare. One could dine at a Mexican restaurant, Italian restaurant, American steakhouse or Japanese grill and the child's menu will not differ: chicken nuggets and fries, macaroni and cheese, hamburger and fries or cheese pizza. Rarely is a salad, vegetable or healthier cut of meat made available, and the meal nearly always comes with a soft drink, so very few families opt for water instead.

In the grocery store, the items marketed towards children are colorful, sugary, highly processed and usually feature a cartoon character on the front. To make a cereal or cracker more appealing to children, artificial colors and unrealistic flavors are often added. Who else would consume a purple or green cheese cracker? Yet, these additives are exactly what children should be avoiding, according to scientific research.

Why are these products marketed towards children? Because it is effective. Children consume artificial "juice" beverages in ridiculous amounts. Birthday parties feature hydrogenated oil laden cupcakes with bright, colorful and sugary frosting. Even childcare centers and church nurseries typically serve cheese crackers (often in bright, unnatural colors), pretzels, wheat crackers, or snack size pouches of cookies or animal crackers - all of which are laden with hydrogenated oil and high fructose corn syrup with the occasional artificial color, flavor and preservative thrown in for good measure.

Yet, without fully understanding the potential effects of their actions, parents continue to purchase these items en masse, prompting manufacturers to continue to roll out new artificial food products. And they will continue to do so as long as parents continue to buy them.

The little known reality is that children can be trained to be just as content with natural, nutrient dense foods, which can often be just as fun as the artificial counterfeits. Even children who are used to the standard childhood diet can learn to love real foods! I've seen it happen and help families accomplish this every day. My tips for making this happen in your home are covered in the next section.

The High Price of "Fun" Foods

What effects do these foods have on our children? Aside from the potential for pesticide and preservative build up, which can lead to chronic life-long health concerns, these manufactured foods can also have immediate health consequences. Many of these health concerns occur so often that we have become to consider them normal phases of childhood, unaware that prevention is even a possibility.

Perhaps the most notable consequence of poor dietary intake among children is the effect these foods have on their cognitive functioning. For individuals whose main job is to spend their days learning how the world works, mastering information that is necessary for future success and exploring new ideas and concepts, these effects can be disastrous, not only for outward success but for internal self evaluation as well. How many students consider themselves to be "bad" at math, or even the entire educational setting, yet when simple dietary changes take place suddenly find themselves able to stay on task, comprehend and analyze the information presented and succeed at tasks previously unattempted? This may be surprising, but it is not uncommon.

The link between food and behavioral problems, developmental delays or other concerns, hyperactivity, concentration and memory is an important one to understand. Due to their rapid development, children's brains are in need of beneficial omega fatty acids, so the intake of hydrogenated oils can be extremely detrimental. When ingested, the half-life of hydrogenated oils is over 50 days, which means today's lunchtime short cut affects their body for months to come.

Newly Common Childhood Disorders

Many of the newer disorders that affect children have been directly linked to diet, and in some cases, have been reversed exclusively by returning to a real foods diet.

Research shows that intake of artificial colors and flavors affects the concentration and attention span of children, and when removed from the diet, many children have seen increases in concentration and, as a result, academic performance. Some cases of diagnosed ADHD have been controlled not with pharmaceuticals but with careful attention to a real foods diet, including the omission of processed, refined and otherwise altered foods. Other children that may require more advanced measures to control their symptoms still typically benefit from a healthier diet, which focuses on brain boosting nutrients and eliminating anything that may inhibit cognitive functioning.

Likewise, many developmental delays can be directly linked to dietary causes, ranging from nutritional deficiencies to inhibition of nutrient utilization by processed foods. Some nutrients, such as iron and zinc, play key roles in typical development, speech delays, and behavioral concerns; overall identifying and treating the deficiency have alleviated developmental delays. Many children with speech delays benefit from omega-3 fatty acid supplements, as they boost the brain's ability to function appropriately, and nutrient dense foods in childhood and even during the pregnancy assist in the prevention of these concerns.

Many parents are aware of the importance of organic baby foods or reducing exposure to harmful substances with newborns in the home, but don't realize that infant health begins not prior to the birth, but prior to conception. The foods a woman consumes from late childhood through the end of her childbearing years play a role, however large or small, in the nutritional availability of a developing baby. Ensuring that nutritional stores are a focus prior to conception is the best way for a new baby to get off to the best start.

Furthermore, many studies now show that some harmful decisions and exposures affect not only the current generation of offspring, but the next 2, 3 or even 4! When a female baby is developing in the womb, so are her reproductive organs and tools. These can be adversely affected by dietary habits of her own mother while still in the womb, but are not apparent in some cases until the baby is grown and her future children have begun to mature.

"Adult" Problems in Children

Another issue that occurs when children consume unhealthy processed foods is the increasing development of so called "adult" disorders in little ones. While 1 in 3 American adults meet the qualifications for obesity, the more shocking numbers are those of our preschoolers. During a time that was historically focused on "fattening" one up, one in seven modern preschoolers are now classified as obese, and many more are overweight. All of the health concerns associated with obesity are present among children, who are facing increased risks of adult onset diabetes and even cardiovascular risks at earlier ages than otherwise common.

Knowing that the longer lifespan allows more and more time for these health concerns to manifest themselves in various ways, the increases rates of obesity, diabetes, cognitive disorders and other dietary related concerns are a problem not to be ignored. The best way to address this is not by counting calories or fat grams, but to focus on healthy, real foods diets, rich in the naturally occurring nutrients children need for optimal health.

Chapter Five: How Did We Get Here?

While the products at the grocery store may be immediately recognizable to modern shoppers as food, our ancestors would have no idea what to do with many, if not most of these items. At no time in history has food changed as much as it has over the last hundred years. Though there were many minor changes in the previous thousands of years, the food trends were relatively consistent. Real foods were consumed. They were consumed with minimal processing. They were consumed without the addition of synthetic chemical compounds for flavor enhancing or preservation. They were consumed from local sources. They were consumed seasonally. Trends came and went. Social classes enjoyed distinct culinary luxuries, but these factors remained constant throughout the years.

Yet, over the last hundred years, we have been removed gradually from the source of our food. While experts place the exact turnaround between 1880 and 1930, the changes continued to increase the distance between the farm and the table and we are more removed from the source of our food than ever. Many schoolchildren don't realize that milk doesn't originate at the grocery store!

These changes could be blamed on government subsidies, advertising executives, public (nutrition based) awareness campaigns, misinformation, the industrialization of food or many other factors, but the reality is that, while each of these factors played key roles, change happens on a personal level. When enough of these individual changes accumulate, nationwide or even worldwide change occurs. So the real question is how did these large factors affect individuals, causing the food industry we have today?

Trendy Foods

When the topic of food history is examined, one prevailing theme can be found, and that is the direct influence culture plays on food selection. Therefore, one could presume that the best way to affect the diet of an entire population is to influence culture, and the earliest nutritional advocates learned this lesson well when their attempts to change the dietary habits of the lower class failed because the lower class was more interested in mimicking the diets of the middle or wealthier classes than it was concerned with foods that were considered to be healthy. To change the diet in America from traditional foods to industry foods required targeting the middle class, who were trying to follow in the footsteps of the wealthy and willing to make any changes and shortcuts necessary for social purposes. When the middle class changed, so did the impoverished.

The wealthy have always generally enjoyed consuming foods that were rare, exotically prepared or altered through an expensive process. This includes refined wheat, a product that has been available to the wealthy since the days of the Pharaohs in ancient Egypt. Processed sugars were prominent in diets of the privileged, as were other expensive ingredients such as fats, oils and prime cuts of meat. Prior to the modern industrial advancements, refining grain was an expensive process and the poor could generally only afford the whole grain or even the items they could grow themselves. Ironically, diets of the poor have traditionally been the healthiest, as expensive sugars, meats and oils were forcibly kept in moderation due to budgetary constraints.

Hence, when the nutrition pioneers determined that whole grain was not the healthiest form of grain and refined wheat was ideal, the population was easily persuaded. When industrial advancements were able to streamline the process of refining grain and expand the industry to cover large areas instead of relying on local resources, many individuals did not see the end of an era of healthy food; they only saw the opportunity to consume the luxurious foods of the wealthy at affordable prices.

More, Bigger, Faster, Better?

With the industrial revolution taking place, the food supply became a quick target. Like everything else, the mantra of "more, bigger, faster" dramatically changed the process of feeding our country. Little family farms began to give way to massive industry farms, which began shipping goods on the newly established railroads. Shipping these goods required preservatives and new methods of agriculture, which quickly hurried to keep up with the growth, happily obliging to the new demands without stopping to consider what the potential consequences of dramatically altering our food supply would be.

Of course, it is easy to argue that, at first, there consequences were minimal. Foods were still considered fresh, little processing was done and everything was "organic" by today's standards. One could even argue that these were beneficial advancements. Suddenly seasonal changes did not exclude the availability of assorted produce. Fresh milk and eggs were available to everyone. This was the beginning of the glory days of food, a time that passed as quickly as it came, leaving many still wondering what happened.

This system evolved over the years to one that relies nearly exclusively on transported food. To transport an annual supply of this food requires more fuel than the average two car family uses in a year. When traveling this far, food loses nutritional value, as it has to be harvested prematurely, and it begins to degrade as it crosses the country or countries.

Not only does food quality suffer under this model, but food safety becomes a serious concern as well. It is difficult to maintain the oversight of such a system, and despite approximately 1/7th of the food supply - 300 million tons of food - being imported into the country annually, inspections are only possible for around 2%. It is practically impossible to put the kind of checks and balances into place that ensure shipment of food, whether domestic or foreign, are free of potential contamination, which could theoretically occur at any time. The risk of illness from food borne pathogens is a very real possibility and the risk of that microbial contamination being resistant to modern treatments is an even scarier, but real concern is due in part to the massive overuse of antibiotics in food meat production. These resistant strands of microbes are difficult and for some, impossible to overcome.

Low Costs and High Productivity

The high volume model of business that was so successful with cars, clothing and other products simply cannot work for food, although that does not stop those that still insist on trying.

While the food system is an economic system, the perishable products of a food system are much more intimate and personal than a pair of jeans or a new car. Living individuals who rely on it to sustain life consume them internally. Contamination is not a concern in a factory assembly line for a new car, but in a food production line, it could be deadly.

Likewise, the massive growth of the food industry is not a sustainable model. Eventually the decision had to be made to continue pursuing quantity or to pull back and retain quality. In our food system, quality died a slow and quiet death. While these decisions are not immediately obvious, with the advantage of hindsight, we can now see where the quality of our food was sacrificed for growth, and the current generation is now paying the price.

Ingredients for food products cannot continue to be treated as typical supplies with the meat and cheese being purchased from the lowest bidder. To maintain these artificially reduced prices, foods are genetically modified, pumped with hormones and antibiotics, and treated with pesticides and fertilizers in the name of uniformity and cost.

Our low cost, high volume model has led to epidemics of obesity, diabetes, heart disease and cancer.

Sustainability

While the current model is neither desirable nor sustainable, the same changes in culture that led to this system can lead the way out. Interestingly enough, the same changes that lead to a more sustainable food supply also lead to a healthier food supply. The system that has worked well for millennia is a system worth repeating.

Despite the health effects of poor quality food and the environmental effects of soil stripping, monoculture and nutrient depletion, these concerns can be corrected, and the food supply still has potential. Many of the modern advancements can be utilized more appropriately to help reduce costs without compromising quality.

These changes include focusing on organic produce, which is more nutrient dense than conventional and restores the soil, leading to continued production of nutrient dense food.

Animal meat production that focuses on grass-fed cattle and free-range chickens is both healthier and more sustainable. The current system requires approximately eight pounds of grain to produce one pound of meat, yet most animals were not even designed to consume grain. Vegetable based diets are also healthier and easier to provide. Limiting meat intake to a more balanced portion of the diet is not difficult and has multiple benefits.

For gardeners and aspiring farmers, the polyculture model ensures continued availability of nutrient dense soil and even helps to provide healthier crops. Large fields of a single crop were not commonplace until recently in history.

Local diets decrease the amount of fuel required to transport produce, limit the nutrient degradation in the food and close the widening gap between the farm and table. Focusing on "slow foods" such as home cooked meals and real foods also eliminates the amount of fuel required to transport our food and ensures that healthy items are prepared without preservatives and additives.

Finally, small and diverse farms, ideally in backyards or neighborhoods, ensures an abundance of healthy, local food and prevents the soil stripping and nutrient loss that is so common among the large, factory farms.

These changes are neither difficult nor challenging, but do require some determination and a willingness to change longstanding habits. However, their implementation ensures a healthy abundant food supply for our children, and inspires the overall growth that changes the eating habits of entire cultures.

Section Two: What to Eat (Identifying Real Foods)

Chapter Six: Criteria for Real Food

Despite the current state of the food industry, most people still believe they are eating real foods. To suggest that the foods available in the grocery store are anything but food is preposterous for most. "*Of course* it is real food," they say, "If it is not real food, then what exactly is it?" Well, these items are edible, and technically they are consumed and digested by humans, which allow them to meet the legal definition for food, but they are nothing like the nourishing, natural foods that our bodies were designed to consume. Many experts call these items "food like substances" because many of the ingredients in store bought foods are unfamiliar to our bodies, and some are downright harmful. The research into the long-term effects of this consumption is frighteningly scarce, and the available good quality nutrition research is overwhelmingly in favor of natural, whole foods.

As we saw in the previous section, consuming these items may continue to keep our bodies alive, but it does not contribute to health, and would hardly be considered the ideal for something we all do three times a day - if not more.

So, what should we consume? What exactly does it mean for a food to be a *real* food? Many authors have created their own food rules or guidelines - many of which are quite good - but most of these lists lead to even more confusion. We've all been told not to consume any food that we can't pronounce, but I've met very few people who can pronounce quinoa, an extremely healthy and inexpensive grain. Likewise, shopping only on the borders of the supermarket assumes that you're shopping a major retailer, which is hardly the place to find high quality local and organic foods at a reasonable price. So, I've established these criteria for real foods for my clients and workshop guests. These are not rules, because my personal philosophy is that food should be focused on what to do, not what not to do. They are simple guidelines. If a food meets most of these guidelines, it is probably a real food.

Where was the food baked / cooked / prepared?

The best place to buy real food is at the bakery, farmer's market or other location that allows you to talk directly to the people making your food. Local bakeries don't need stabilizers or preservatives to maintain freshness, because they are selling the bread to the consumer (you) the same day it is baked. Foods purchased where they were prepared or directly from the person who prepared them are more likely to actually be real foods.

Of course, this can be tricky, as it appears that fast food is cooked on location, but the reality is that their deliveries are not of ingredients, but items that have been prepared and frozen at a large factory miles away. They are merely reheating the food in most cases, not actually cooking it. Cooking requires more than merely applying heat to an item. Cooking includes measuring and preparing ingredients, assembling them together, and concludes with applying heat. Most restaurants sweep in for the final step and present the product as though it were homemade.

Another way to ask this question is, "Who devised the recipe for this item?" Local bakeries and farmers typically serve recipes handed down from parents or grandparents, or those they created themselves. High quality eateries have trained chefs in the kitchen that design restaurant specific specialties with the best ingredients they can find. If you can't ask the chef what went into an item, chances are that it came pre-packaged. In some extreme cases, you can't even customize a menu item because it is pre-assembled before arriving at the restaurant.

Real foods are cooked and prepared by real people, who take pride in their work and sell it directly to the person / people who will consume or serve the product.

Do you recognize the ingredients?

If the item is in a grocery store or market and has an ingredient list, glance through it. When you read the contents, can you mentally picture the ingredients? If it contains flour, we all know what a bowl of flour looks like, and where it came from. If it contains modified food starch, what does that look like and where did it come from? Real foods are made with real ingredients. Real foods and real ingredients are made in kitchens, not laboratories.

Of course, some ingredients may be new. Quinoa is an example I like to use. It is unfamiliar to many people, but extremely healthy. Yet, when most people see the word *quinoa,* they know it is a grain or bean or vegetable or something that grew somewhere out of the ground - again, not in the laboratory. In other words, you should have some idea, even if it is vague, of where the food came from.

In most cases, the name of the food will be very telling as to its origins. Ingredients with words like modified, hydrogenated, artificial, hydrolyzed and anything that has numbers following it are not real foods and did not come from a farm, a yard, a bakery or anywhere else real foods comes from.

Does the item look like something you've seen in nature?

Likewise, the item or ingredients should resemble textures and colors you've seen in nature. Bright blue candies with thick shells are not found in nature. Neither are hot pink crackers. While natural foods come in a variety of shapes, textures and colors, they are all (usually) recognizable. Strawberries, cherries and raspberries are bright red. Beans are usually hues of brown and green. Citrus fruits usually come in colors with yellow in them. And so on.

The food, and more importantly, the ingredients, should resemble shapes, colors and textures that are found in nature. Of course, there are always surprises. Red lentils are actually a shade of orange that resembles neon, but their texture, shape and taste give away their true identity.

Check the color, texture, shape and any other details of the item and ingredient list. If you can't possibly imagine them in nature, chances are, they probably didn't come from nature. Look for something else.

Could you make this in a well-stocked home kitchen, given the time and talent?

The purpose of purchasing prepared food is to save time and enjoy the talents of others. Otherwise, everything can and should be made at home. If you don't have the time to grow, harvest and grind wheat, then bake it into bread, you buy a loaf from a baker. This practice is not new and would definitely qualify as traditional. Older cities had bakers, millers and other occupations that helped provide shortcuts for meal planning and preparation. Yet, over time, it appears we have forgotten the purpose of purchasing food.

We don't purchase food because we don't have the processing equipment at home to make our own hydrogenated oils and crackers of a uniform sized and shape. We purchase them because we are busy or because maybe our cracker baking skills are not the best. Whatever the reason, it is not because we *can't* bake a loaf of bread or a batch of crackers at home.

Therefore, any real foods available at a market or grocery store will be items we have the ability to produce at home. If you look at an item and wonder, "How in the world did they make this?" It's probably not a real food.

If you did make this food at home, how long would it last?

A homemade loaf of bread will typically become stale in 3-5 days. If baker's yeast was used, it will begin to grow mold in less than a week under normal circumstances. If the bread was baked in a factory on the other side of the country, shipped to your local grocer and spent a day or two on their shelves before you purchased it, how long should it last?

Natural preservation techniques such as canning, drying and freezing help foods to last longer. Contrary to popular belief, foods in the frozen section are typically much fresher and contain fewer (if any) preservatives than those available in the refrigerated section of a store. Unless the food was prepared in that store and placed in the cooler within days of purchase, it requires a large amount of preservatives to prevent contamination.

Interestingly enough, many techniques to remove the individuality of real foods actually decrease their shelf life. For example, unwashed farm fresh eggs can last many months under refrigeration, but store bought eggs have a dramatically reduced shelf life due to the washing solutions designed to make the products appear tidy and uniform. Likewise, real bread does not usually grow mold; it becomes stale and dry. Dried bread can often be "revived" with some water and a short trip to the oven. Bread baked with baker's yeast, however, grows mold and cannot be salvaged. These oddities are due to the natural microbial balance within foods that protect and preserve them from dangerous pathogens. When we tamper with a system that works, it usually ends up worse, not better.

So, how to tell if the food should be stable or perishable? Generally speaking, fresh, real, raw ingredients should be fairly stable. Preparing the food reduces the shelf life and should be consumed quickly.

How long has this food been a part of the human diet?

Have you ever read a history book that talks about breakfast cereals in the days of the pioneers? Or visited a history museum to watch the re-enactors open a package of gummy candy for their children, then bake a tube of biscuits? Of course not. Without the option to choose from various food imitations, previous generations - with the exception of the most recent, which got us into this mess - consumed only local, real foods. Not for their health, but out of necessity. There were no other options.

Therefore, a quick and easy way to determine if a food is a real food or not is to picture it in a pioneer village — or an ancient Egyptian or Roman town — any setting that existed prior to the mass adulteration of food. If doing that makes you giggle, chances are it is not a real food. If it fits the scenario, it's real.

Over a thousand new foods hit the shelves each year. Many of these are nothing more than rearrangements of the same thing, and most of them are lacking nutritionally. While some (though very few) of them may be fine for consumption, it is quite hard to improve on the natural ingredients already available.

Chapter Seven: How To Recognize Real Foods

One of the biggest hindrances to consuming real foods is the sneaky advertising and marketing that many food manufacturers get away with. This confuses the consumer, causing many individuals to purchase items thinking they are natural or healthy, when in fact, they contain hydrogenated oils, artificial colors or flavors or other additives. The best way to avoid this is learning how to recognize and identify real foods. This habit takes a little practice, and the first trip to the grocery store may take much longer than normal, but after just a few trips, you'll be a pro at distinguishing between real foods and counterfeits.

The first thing to realize is that most claims on a label are intentionally vague, utilizing loopholes found in lax regulations to help foods appear healthier than they are. Terms like *natural* may not mean anything at all, and even more definite terms like *trans-fat free* don't mean what many people think they mean. Natural may be the most confusing advertising term, as it implies that the foods is, well, natural. Unfortunately, *natural* is subjective and is not regulated by any authority. In other words, if I want to claim my new cracker made with corn syrup, margarine and white sugar is natural, nobody will stop me. It is most popular among meat producers, who advertise that their meat is natural. This may seem like a good buy, but natural meat tells nothing of the growth conditions, the animal feed, the treatment of the animal or the medicinal history of the animal. In other words, a conventionally raised animal could produce natural meat.

If so many claims are confusing, is it necessary to memorize all of them, testing yourself at each trip to the supermarket? Not at all. Everything you need to know is provided on the side of the container, in a box better known as the nutrition label. This label offers quite a bit of information of the true health of a food, but few individuals actually know how to read it.

Most people flip the product over to the label, glance at the total fat content, the total carb content and perhaps the total calories and make a decision based off that. These few classifications tell little to nothing about the nutrient content of the food.

First, counting calories, carbohydrates or fat grams is not the way to achieve health - or weight loss, for that matter. Consuming real foods diets, with plenty of variety and in moderate amounts, combined with lifestyle changes such as increased exercise is what will result in healthy, lasting weight loss.

Next, even if it was a good idea to count the carbohydrate, calorie or fat content of a food, without looking at serving sizes, the numbers on the box mean nothing. What if the serving size is actually about 1/4 of what you typically consume? In many cases, that is exactly the case. Many single serving sized bags of chips, pretzels or drinks actually contain 2-4 servings, according to the label. So, any numbers you read on the side need to be doubled, tripled or more, based on your idea of a serving.

Furthermore, the idea of counting calories, carbohydrates and fat grams is based on outdated ideas, which are not rooted in good science. When I teach classes on real foods, the most important concept I try to get across is to look not at the box, but below it. Beneath the nutritional facts box is where the most valuable information about a food product can be found. This is where you will find the ingredient list.

On the ingredient list, any claims found on the front of the box will be verified or discarded. This list includes every ingredient that can be found in the product (with exceptions for small and / or indirect additives) and they are listed in order, based upon volume. If sugar is the predominant ingredient in the food, sugar will be first on the list. If hydrogenated oils have been used, the oil will be identified as hydrogenated. Furthermore, you can discover every single type of sugar, grain, oil or substance that will be found in the food inside.

This allows you to examine the oil content, not based upon how much oil will be present in a serving, but on what type of oil is found in this food. It enables you to discover what types of grains have been used, and how they were processed prior to their inclusion in the product. The exact type of sugar can be uncovered, enabling you to consider how that sugar will impact your body or your child's body - not merely how much unidentified sugar is in the product.

From this information, you can evaluate the food based upon how it will really affect the body, knowing that not all fats are equal, not all carbohydrates are equal and not all calories are equal. After this examination, if you or a family member has a health concern that requires consideration of the total number of sugar grams or fat grams, you can check the total grams per serving - and consider the serving size - knowing not only how many grams are in the serving, but what quality those grams represent. Of course, for most real foods, this should not come as a surprise. A box of cookies or jar of fruit preserves typically has more grams of sugar than a loaf of bread. Likewise, a container of ice cream will usually have more fat than a carton of yogurt. Once the ingredients have been determined to be healthy, and present in an ideal ratio (i.e. the flour is listed *before* the sugar), then the total counts should just be a verification, not a surprise.

Reading the Ingredient List

While reading the ingredient list, a few basic principles apply. First, remembering the criteria for real food, look through the list and see how familiar the ingredients are. Do they sound like a garden or bulk foods product list? Or do they sound like something from a chemistry class you took in school? Generally speaking, most words should be easily recognizable, and if you can't pronounce them, it shouldn't be because they have 4-5 syllables.

Look for red flags such as hydrogenated, hydrolyzed, artificial, anything with a number following it, modified, processed and anything similar. Avoid these in favor of real food ingredients such as flour, oats, salt, etc.

Some store bought prepared foods will need a preservative. If that is the case, learn about these items and know which preservatives or additives you are comfortable with your family eating. The resources section at the end of this book has brief descriptions of the most common additives.

Once the artificial or processed ingredients are reduced or eliminated, focus on high quality whole foods ingredients. Many ingredients have tricky names, which allow them to appear to be something they are not. The best way to identify these is to pay close attention to the exact wording on the label.

For example, *wheat flour* appears to be a healthy, whole grain - a perfect addition to the diet. But, if you pay attention, it did not say *whole*-wheat flour, only wheat flour. We often falsely associate the word *wheat* with whole wheat because of the common "white or wheat" question. The reality is that both flours come from wheat. In this example, the word wheat merely identifies which grain the flour came from - it does not imply that the flour is whole, not refined. If the ingredient list does not contain *whole-wheat flour,* then the flour is more than likely refined.

Other tricky ingredients include those with explanations beside them. While many explanations are regulated and required for the additive, some include language that is vague. This includes substances such as natural sweetener, natural emulsifier, or even derived from corn or soy, which implies that the substance is a mere extract, not a processed ingredient. Typically, these terms are not reliable, as the terminology is used with little oversight and no real meaning.

Reading the ingredient list is also important because it identifies substances that may be able to, through loopholes, not appear elsewhere on the labeling. One great example of this is trans fatty acids and hydrogenated oils. Technically, a product can claim to contain 0 trans fats as long as a serving contains less than 0.5 grams. Many serving sizes are much smaller than what is actually consumed by the average individual. If each cookie contained 0.4 grams trans fatty acids, the box could legally claim to be trans fat free. Yet, eating 4 of these cookies would provide nearly 2 grams of trans fatty acids.

However, these fats are a byproduct of the hydrogenation process. If the label claims to be free of trans fatty acids, but the ingredient list includes hydrogenated or partially hydrogenated oils, the item is not truly trans fat free. Any label claiming "0 grams *trans* fats," "*trans* fat free," or "not a significant source of *trans* fatty acids" may legally contain up to 0.5 grams per serving. The acceptable intake of trans fatty acids is zero, however. This is a very common marketing ploy, and the same labeling guideline applies to other types of fats including total fat content and saturated fat content.

Claims of Nutritional Content

While the loopholes may give the appearance that a food manufacturer can place anything they like on the package, the actual guidelines are quite strict. Labeling a food product is a careful process with standards set in some cases for even the permissible type size and font. While the rules are quite broad and have many specifics, the general guidelines do not allow any item to use the words "free," "zero," "without," "no, trivial source of" or "dietary insignificant source of" if there is more than 0.5 grams of the substance per serving.

"Little," "low," and "few" are only permissible if the calorie content is below 40, if the fat content is below 3 grams, if the saturated fat is below 1 gram and if the sodium is below 140 mg. However, specific requirements may vary for individual foods. The words "reduced," "less," "lower" and "fewer" should contain at least 25% less of the substance than similar or reference foods.

Some of these modifications may simply be the result of different preparation methods or better ingredients. For example, an item that is usually fried may be baked to result in reduced fat. Likewise, many fat free items are naturally fat free. However, many items with reduced or eliminated fat or calories have been modified and processed further to result in this claim. These modifications are often based on trends in diet and nutrition, and have historically been disastrous.

At the Store

The best way to identify real foods is to ignore the claims on the front of the package. Ignore the box counting individual fat grams or calories. Ignore any pre-conceived ideas about the health benefits, or lack thereof, of any food, and look at the ingredient list. Identify the ingredients and determining if they are processed, modified or naturally occurring. Remember that the ingredients are listed in order, by weight. If sugar, (even naturally occurring sugar) is the first ingredient, the product will be high in sugar. From there, if health needs or preferences dictate watching sugar content or fat content, after establishing that the sugars and fats present are acceptable forms of the nutrient, move back up to the top of the box and evaluate the total numbers to see if they are acceptable amounts for your unique preferences or needs.

Chapter Eight: Seven Confusing Foods

Once we embark on the journey to real, healthy and natural foods, we inevitably reach those certain items that seem to confuse just about everyone. The food rules abound, with many insisting everyone should avoid red meat, milk, fish, bread and so on. Then, others insist that red meat, milk, fish or bread should be a central part of a healthy diet. Which is it? How can anyone ever be sure? While the science of nutrition is still in its infancy, with great strides over the last century and during that time, the most common lesson learned is that the natural balance existed for a purpose.

In this chapter, I will examine seven of the most confusing foods (bread, grains, meat, milk, oils, seafood, sweeteners) identifying the known research, the traditional role in the diet, the health aspects and, of course, my thoughts on the subject. I think you'll be happy to find that many of them are not quite as confusing as they initially appear, and the information is fairly easy to understand and apply to real life!

Bread: The notion that bread is anything but a health food may have seemed comical to the ancients, provided we first explained our concepts of health foods to them, of course! Yet, I also highly doubt any of them would have recognized the bizarre substances sold in our grocery stores that pass for bread. When many families make the change to healthier, natural foods, the idea of bread is examined closely. The type of flour often changes from refined, bleached, white flour to organic whole-wheat flour, often freshly ground right in the kitchen to preserve the maximum nutrient quantity. This is then combined with fresh water, sea salt and a packet of baker's yeast to produce a healthy loaf of nourishing bread. It seems quite simple, right? Fresh flour, water, salt, maybe some local honey and of course the packet of natural yeast. But - just how natural is that packet of yeast? And, if this bread is the staff of life referred to throughout history, why do so many people have trouble with its digestion and metabolization, or even benefiting from its nutrient content? Perhaps something is amiss.

The bread that supported our ancestors looked nothing like even the homemade bread produced in a healthy, natural kitchen, for several reasons. We're going to discuss the two most critical differences, and then we'll see why modern bread may not be a health food, but real bread is definitely a nutritional must-have.

The first difference in bread is a variable that changes throughout time and across cultures - the type of flour. Most modern bread features one type of flour, wheat. Occasionally other flours may be added as flavoring, but their content rarely exceeds 10-15% of the overall content. Consumption of wheat far exceeds other grains in most diets, primarily because of this fact. However, our ancestors often consumed a wide variety of grains in their breads. In fact, barley was often the grain consumed by the poor, and it was not uncommon to bake breads that were mixtures of many grains, beans and legumes. While wheat or barley may have been the featured grain in most cases, they were not as exclusive as they are in modern diets. This little notion makes a big nutritional difference.

Wheat provides many important nutrients, including vitamins, minerals, healthy carbohydrates and protein. Yet, other grains offer complementing nutrients and when combined either in the same loaf or in the same individual's diet, the result is an improved and expanded nutritional intake with a variety of essential amino acids, proteins, vitamins, minerals and more.

Additionally, modern wheat does not have the same composition previous wheat had. Wheat has been bred to contain higher amounts of gluten, the protein matrix that allows the bread to grow, holding the air bubbles produced by the growing yeast. This allows bread to be soft and fluffy. However, many individuals cannot tolerate gluten for numerous health reasons. Many children with special needs or behavioral concerns find dramatic improvement when gluten is removed from the diet, even temporarily, and many children and adults have celiac disease, which is a lifelong intolerance to gluten. These health concerns are relatively new, and rapidly growing in number, causing many to wonder what happened.

So, how can this be corrected? Fairly easily: simply strive for a variety of flours and grains in the breads you bake and purchase. This results in a varied intake of nutrients that can help boost the nutritional stores of many different compounds within the body.

The next difference is not quite as apparent at first glance. While yeast has raised loaves of bread for millennia, the baker's yeast available in grocery stores today is an unnatural yeast, specifically bred to hasten and streamline the baking process. While that slight adjustment may seem to be harmless, further study reveals otherwise.

Throughout history, until the last hundred years, yeast was obtained directly from the air. Flour and water were left out to collect the natural leaven present in the air, and the yeasts and bacteria grew in the substance, causing it to rise, forming what we recognize as a loaf of bread. With the advancement of microbial understanding, scientists were able to isolate specific strands of yeast and breed new strands, which are not found in nature. One of these new strands, *Saccharomyces cerevisiae,* better known as baker's yeast, completely changed the baking process. Instead of relying on weather, skill and other unpredictable factors, baking could be streamlined, producing uniform loaves in specific timeframes. This advancement changed the microbial blend of multiple yeast strands and bacterial strands to a single type of yeast, often added to the dough in abnormally large amounts when compared to the natural fermentation process.

While the improvement may have seemed innocent, these changes affected the quality of the bread and its nutritional value. Naturally fermented bread inhibits the phytic acid found in wheat. Phytic acid inhibits the bioavailability of iron, magnesium and zinc, three extremely common nutrient deficiencies in the modern diet. Despite conventional bread appearing to contain a healthy supply of iron, zinc and magnesium, research shows that it can actually deplete the body of these nutrients, whereas naturally leavened bread increases the bioavailability of these important substances.

Naturally fermented bread also has a lower glycemic index, meaning that it is a healthier choice for balanced diets as it does not contribute to the typical highs and lows of refined carbohydrate consumption. I'm sure these nutritional differences played a key role in bread falling from the "staff of life" to the indulgent junk food it is today.

Grains: These foods are dense sources of many nutrients and are a cheap source of calories for feeding the world. Few would argue their nutritional value, but many confuse poor quality grains with nutrient rich grains, eventually causing grains to be wrongly classified as harmful among some fad diets. This is easily remedied by looking for whole, unprocessed grains.

Most seeds of grain contain three key parts: the endosperm, the germ and the bran. The endosperm composes around 80-85% of the grain and is composed primarily of starch and protein. While these are important elements, the grain stores the B vitamins, minerals and much of the fiber elsewhere. The germ is a mere 3% of the grain and is rich in vitamin E. The outer bran, roughly 15% of the grain, contains most of the fiber and the other nutrients such as B vitamins and zinc. In refined flour, the bran and germ are removed, taking their important nutrients with them.

Grains provide valuable fiber to the diet, which results in many health benefits including reduced risks of colon cancer, constipation, hemorrhoids, gallstones, high cholesterol, ulcers and various heart conditions. Grains also add protein to the diet, but it is important to remember that the proteins are not *complete* proteins. In other words, they provide some, but not all of the essential amino acids we need for survival.

Ancient cultures generally understood this and complemented grains with legumes or beans, which typically contain matching incomplete amino acids. Together, complete proteins are formed. While some would insist that this combining take place at a single meal, our bodies were fearfully and wonderfully made, and they know how to handle the proteins as they come. Food combining at the same meal or even the same day is not necessary.

The primary concern with grains is the poor quality commonly available, and the confusion surrounding the distinction between poor quality and high quality grains. So, let's look at a few. **Barley** is one of the oldest grains and is somewhat similar to wheat. It is somewhat rich in gluten, though it contains less than wheat, grows well in many climates and is extremely versatile. Barley offers many minerals, B vitamins, fiber and medicinal properties, particularly benefiting digestion. Pearled barley is easier to cook, but offers fewer nutrients than whole barley.

Buckwheat is actually a thistle, not a grass. It produces groats, which are fruits, encased in a shell, but does not contain bran and germ like other grains. However, its nutritional profile, which is similar to most grains, and its flavor generally cause it to be considered a grain. Whole buckwheat is healthy offering many minerals and B vitamins. It can be used as a flour and mixed with other grains.

Corn is actually a true grain, but can be consumed as a vegetable. While it offers many nutritional benefits, the genetic modification of the grain coupled with its widespread, somewhat uninhibited growth, have caused it to fall into disrepute. Corn is a great source of B vitamins and minerals and organic corn is GMO free, and can be a part of a healthy diet. However, many corn products are of suspect health because they have been refined or processed.

Millet is another ancient grain with a bountiful B vitamin content. It is gluten free and one of the most alkaline grains, which means it is less likely to lead to congestion. It cooks quickly and easily, making it a perfect whole grain addition to any meal.

Quinoa is another "grain" that is technically not a grain but is generally consumed as one. It is rich in protein and contains every essential amino acid, which is rare for a non-meat protein. Most cultures that heavily rely on grains for protein become deficient in lysine because it is rare in grains. Quinoa, however, contains all amino acids, including lysine. It cooks quickly and is a great addition to cookie dough, rice, pasta dishes, salads, or on its own with some herbs and seasonings.

Rice is a grain that has come under fire lately, as most rice is refined, white rice, not nutritious brown rice. However, rice is the primary staple food for a whopping two thirds of the world. In many countries, the average annual rice consumption is 100 pounds per person. As a complex carbohydrate, rice provides plenty of energy in the diet. It also offers fiber, which aids in healthy digestion, and an assortment of B vitamins.

Rice can also provide iron, protein, calcium, phosphorus and potassium. It is also just as famous for what it does not have, which includes gluten, cholesterol, sodium and fat.

Rice has a natural hull surrounding it for protection, but this hull is inedible, so it must be removed. The differences in how rice is processed from this point are outlined in this excerpt from the *World's Healthiest Foods* website:

> "The process that produces brown rice removes only the outermost layer, the hull, of the rice kernel and is the least damaging to its nutritional value. The complete milling and polishing that converts brown rice into white rice destroys 67%

of the vitamin B3, 80% of the vitamin B1, 90% of the vitamin B6, half of the manganese, half of the phosphorus, 60% of the iron, and all of the dietary fiber and essential fatty acids. Fully milled and polished white rice is required to be "enriched" with vitamins B1, B3 and iron."

Obviously, brown rice is the best source of nutrients. White rice, like other refined foods, should not be considered to be an acceptable alternative. There are plenty of alternatives for whole rice that can be adjusted to suit any dish. Many add color, flavor and texture such as basmati, Arborio, black, pecan, red, and others.

The last grain I will cover is the ever-so-common wheat. While many individuals cannot consume the gluten in wheat, those who can will benefit from its impressive nutritional profile. Wheat is an ancient grain that forms the base of nearly all-modern day breads. Like rice, it is a key source of nutrients, as an estimated 1/3 of the world's population depends on wheat for nourishment. Whole wheat (note the word "whole") offers B complex vitamins, protein, manganese, fiber, tryptophan and vitamin E.

Wheat is generally available in a couple of forms, although there are literally thousands of potential varieties. Hard wheat has a higher gluten content, making it ideal for breads. Soft wheat is lower in gluten, making it more suitable for pastries and cakes. Wheat is also named for the season in which it was sown. Spring wheat is sown in the spring and harvested in the fall, offering a higher gluten content. Winter wheat is generally sown in the fall, germinates, and then grows in the spring. This process usually makes winter wheat richer in minerals.

Meat: This is another one of those foods that are confusing, primarily because of the misinformation that abounds. While it is definitely true that a plant-based diet is ideal, this does not necessarily exclude consumption of meat in a healthy diet. In reality, meat can be extremely beneficial for many individuals, provided that the intake is a balanced part of the diet and the meat is healthy.

Conventional meat is often raised on antibiotics and hormones to cut corners wherever possible. This results in lower costs at the grocery store, but comes at a great cost to the consumer's health. Chickens are raised in record numbers of days, and are grown so quickly that their bodies cannot develop in time to properly hold their own weight. They are confined in close quarters and are not able to become healthy. If the animal is not healthy, how can its meat be healthy?

Cows are also raised with numerous additives, including foods that their stomachs were not designed to consume, with the intention of hastening the butchering process and producing more meat in record time. In other words, animal meat production has been streamlined factory style, as if the process of raising an animal has room for improvement. It doesn't.

By confining the animals in ridiculously close quarters, feeding them foods they were not designed to consume, and hurrying them to the butcher, we have successfully adulterated meat to the point that it is no longer healthy or safe.

Cows that are not grass fed contain far more omega 6 fatty acids and far fewer nutritional benefits than cows that are raised on grass. Additionally, cows that are confined in close quarters and fed grain are more likely to be carriers of pathogenic bacteria and microbes such as *E coli* 0157:H7, a potentially fatal and highly resistant strand of *E coli*.

Yet, research shows that cows that roam freely and consume grass are much less likely to carry pathogenic microbes, and that taking a cow out of conventional confinement and dietary habits and placing it in a field of grass can successfully cleanse it of the microbes, eliminating the health risks of the meat.

The routine use of antibiotics with cattle is another concern with potential human health risks. Researchers have found that resistant strains exist for the types of antibiotics used in cattle that are not approved for human use. The World Health Organization has deemed antibiotic resistant bacteria to be one of the most pressing issues of our day, yet antibiotics are continually being overused in both conventional medical settings and conventional farm settings.

Oddly enough, countries that have restricted or banned the routine use of antibiotics in cattle have found that the cost difference is extremely minor and that the process is easy to adapt. Further more, they have found that antibiotics in a medical setting are much more effective, and that some antibiotic resistant strains of disease have virtually disappeared from the population.

The best way to consume meat is to look for farmers and meat processors that are passionate about providing healthy meat. I personally visit the farm that raises my family's meat and can see the conditions in which the animals are raised. I know what their definition of "free range" is, what the animals consume on a day-to-day basis, how they are kept and how they are processed when the time comes.

While learning about the origins of the meat on your table may not be initially as appealing as learning about the origins of the tomato, the safety and health of your family may benefit from a little additional curiosity into the history of your meats.

Milk: This is probably one of the most confusing foods we consume. The question of whether or not milk is a healthy drink for human adults is hotly debated, and assuming that it is, the type of milk ideally consumed opens a whole new debate. While there are no definitive answers that are perfect for everyone, there are some important considerations regarding this milk debate.

The first question is whether or not milk is a healthy food. For some, this may seem to be a no-brainer. Our current culture aside, fresh liquid milk from a cow or goat has not always been a primary part of the human diet. Humans are the only mammals to consume milk from another species, and while fresh animal milk was occasionally consumed by our ancestors, the more common method of consuming animal milk was through fermented drinks, such as kefir and something similar to what we would call yogurt. For young children, breastmilk consumption was the norm through about 4 years of age (possibly older, depending on the specific culture and the source). Babies that could not be breastfed were nursed by another human, and this modern concept that young children need animal milk is a relatively new one.

Is milk a bad thing? Not necessarily. It does contain many nutrients, including protein and fat. However, it also contains certain types of protein that are very difficult for the human body, especially a young one, to digest. It also contains sugars that cause reactions in many individuals and various substances that are generally mucus forming in most individual. In children, a milk sensitivity is one of the most common causes of recurring ear infections and skin conditions such as eczema among clients I have worked with. Eliminating dairy from the diet often relieves many inflammatory conditions and sensitivity related or allergic conditions.

Just as the natural fermentation altered the type of protein in the naturally leavened bread, a fermented milk beverage, such as yogurt or kefir, contains altered proteins that are more easily digested. They also contain beneficial or "friendly" bacteria, which further aid in digestion. These products are good alternatives for those who cannot tolerate liquid milk but feel dairy is an important part of the diet.

The decision of whether or not to consume milk is a personal one. It is easy to consume a healthy diet without it, contrary to what the commercials may suggest. However, if it appears to be tolerated well, there is nothing wrong with adding it to the diet, either.

Including it in the diet brings about an entirely new set of concerns, specifically, what kind of milk is ideal? Should it be fresh, raw milk from a local farmer? Pasteurized, homogenized milk from the grocery store? Organic? Should it even come from a cow? All great questions, and again, there is no one right answer.

Raw milk is milk that has not been through the process of homogenization and pasteurization. While homogenization is an appearance issue, the pasteurization is the aspect that is debatable. There are valid safety arguments on both sides of the debate - namely that pasteurization kills all bacteria, eliminating the benefits of the good bacteria, which work to keep pathogenic bacteria at bay. However, there are also documented cases of transmission of pathogenic bacteria to humans through the intake of raw cow milk. The issue revolves around the health of the cow and the hygienic practices of the individual obtaining the milk from the cow. These are extremely important issues for anyone who chooses raw cow milk to consider. My personal recommendation is that pregnant women, children younger than about 5-7 (depending on size and health) and the elderly don't consume raw milk unless they (or the individual responsible for feeding them) are extremely knowledgeable on the topic, are certain of the cow's health and living conditions and have personally milked the cow.

Otherwise, pasteurized, but non-homogenized milk is a good option, though fermented milk products would be even better as they provide the healthy bacteria often found in raw milk.

Another decision to make is what type of milk. While cow milk is the most common currently, it has not always been that way. Nutritionally, goat's milk is far superior to cow's milk, especially for children. It contains far more nutrients than cow's milk, with only two exceptions, both of which are minor differences. It also contains proteins that are quite similar to breast milk, meaning they are easily digested even for those with sensitive tummies. Goat's milk also lends itself nicely to fermented dairy beverages, highlighting the nutritional benefits while easing the digestive process.

Oils: With few exceptions, most oils are liquid fats obtained from vegetable sources, while most "fats" are solid oils obtained from animal sources. The saturation is what determines whether an oil is solid or liquid, and coconut, palm and palm kernel oil are the rare saturated fats from vegetable sources. Common unsaturated fats include almond, avocado, peanut, corn, olive, safflower, sesame, soybean and sunflower. Olive oil, a monounsaturated fat, is suitable for cooking, while the other oils should not be heated as heat affects the chemical structure, causing the body to have difficulty processing the oil. While cold pressed oils are more costly, they are superior for this reason as well. In addition to not being heated, they were extracted without the use of solvents, which can increase the potential for indirect additives, mainly toxins.

The subject of oils can be quite confusing, but my personal rule is to only use unsaturated oils for room temperature foods or for quick cooking items. For sustained high heat, I use safflower oil, which can tolerate the heat, or a saturated fat, which would not be prone to oxidation. Fresh, cold pressed oils are always ideal, and as with anything, the less processing, refining and altering, the better.

Seafood: Seafood played a key role in the traditional Mediterranean diet, but modern problems with pollution have led many types of seafood to become unsafe and the confusion has caused many to avoid it altogether. This is unfortunate, as fish are ideal foods, rich in nutrients and moderate amounts of healthy fats. The protein in fish is high quality and easily usable by the body.

Fish can and should be an important part of a healthy, real foods diet. Many professionals believe that consuming fish 2-3 times a week helps to reduce the risk of heart disease due to the beneficial fats. Fish also provide the important omega 3 fatty acids that so many of us are deficient in. The fats in fish are healthy fats that prevent disease. Fish is also rich in vitamins and minerals, especially vitamins A and D.

Shellfish, however, are not the ideal types of fish for nutritional benefits. Mollusks such as clams, oysters and scallops are likely to contain concentrated pollutants from the seawater in their bodies, as they are the garbage cans of the sea. These pollutants include not only heavy metals but also contamination from sewage, toxins and PCBs.

Crustaceans are not as big of a concern for toxin accumulation but are still not as healthy as other types of fish. The guide to fish in the back of this book covers some of the healthier, pollutant free varieties of fish.

Sweeteners: Sugar is bad. Or, that is the theory at least. However, that notion is primarily due to the commonality of refined, white sugar as an abundant part of the diet. While that may be the case, not all sweeteners are bad, assuming they are used as a balanced part of a healthy diet.

Historically, sugar was something that was expensive and difficult to obtain. It was treasured and used on special occasions.

Families didn't dump two cups into breakfast muffins, then two more cups into some cookies after school and two cups into dinner or dessert. It was rationed.

While some refined sugars may have been available, more common was the use of maple syrup, honey or ground sugarcane. This difference is crucial, as the natural sugars contain many nutrients that are necessary to their processing within the body. To metabolize and digest sugars, certain nutrients are required. If the sugar itself does not supply those nutrients, the body must rob itself to process what has been put into it. Everything we put into our bodies requires a response. By robbing from ourselves, we set ourselves up for insulin resistance, obesity and other health concerns related to the over-consumption of refined sugars.

Natural sugars, however, generally provide the necessary nutrients for their digestion and metabolism. By doing this, they are more easily processed by the body and won't lead to the problems we tend to associate with consumption of sweeteners.

Of course, this does not mean that natural sugars can be consumed in large quantities. Again looking back at traditional diets for guidance, sweeteners were rare and limited in use. Instead, naturally sweet foods such as fruits were used to satisfy a sweet tooth, serve as dessert or sweeten up breakfast. By following those examples, we can sneak in some additional healthy fruits, which are both sweet and full of nutrients such as vitamins, minerals and fiber, and we can reduce our dependence on concentrated sweeteners.

Then, as appropriate, natural sweetening options are available for special occasions and celebrations and provide the body the nutrients necessary for their safe consumption.

Section Three: How to Eat (Making The Change)

Chapter Nine: Getting There From Here

Changing the entire family's diet from a conventional one to one filled with real foods is often met with resistance, and usually leaves the parent initiating the change overwhelmed, confused and frustrated. After learning just how bad the modern diet is, and how many changes need to be made, it is tempting to try to do it all at once. In my experience, families that take this approach often end up emptying the pantry and fridge, filling it with expensive and exotic ingredients, getting frustrated with the recipes and new preparation methods, then ordering pizza.

There is a better way!

Changing the diet of the entire family involves not only consuming different foods, but also establishing new shopping habits, new cooking methods, investing more time and sometimes even requiring new kitchenware. These are not things that can or should happen overnight; instead they should be the result of a gradual lifestyle change. Remember, you may have been eating this way for 20, 30 or even 40 plus years! Many children may not know any other way of eating and many adults have never really consumed whole foods regularly. These major lifestyle changes are beneficial and are easy to adapt, but they are changes, and any change requires a little determination and even some stubbornness!

I recommend making a plan with specific goals identified, complete with dates to achieve each goal. This helps get some momentum going, as you can always look back at how far you've come, and it enables the family to come together with a common goal. These goals can be as big or little as you choose, but they must be specific, they must have realistic steps in place to be achieved, and they must be workable. Set both short-term goals and long-term goals, and if you've got children on board, setting some fun rewards when certain goals are met is a great way to keep them involved. Great ideas include a cooking class, attempting a new, difficult recipe or even a fun family picnic at a favorite getaway. Here are some additional tips to get started.

Start Small

Rome wasn't built in a day, and anything worth working for will take some time to get right. When people come to learn about the major concerns with the typical food system, they tell me about heading to the grocery store to find it is no longer filled with cereal, snacks and drinks. Instead, they can find nothing but high fructose corn syrup, hydrogenated oils and artificial colors! Where did the food go? Often leaving frustrated after an hour or two of finding nothing suitable for the family to eat, the path to a healthier diet reaches its first main roadblock, and *overwhelmed* becomes an understatement.

This feeling is completely understandable, and quite common. The desire to change has set in, but the taste buds, eating habits and cooking habits have yet to catch up. Instead of trying to change everything right out of the gate, I recommend prioritizing the changes and working on them one or two at a time. Choose what affects your family the most, whether it is high fructose corn syrup, conventional meats, preservatives or hydrogenated oils. Start there, master the change, and then work towards the next goal.

This allows the family to slowly adjust to the new habit, and removes much of the guilt and frustration that occurs with an overnight change in the pantry. Sure, it allows certain habits to continue longer than you may want them to, but the changes you make one at a time are longer lasting and more permanent than overnight makeovers, which are generally met with resistance. I recommend picking a goal that is easy to meet, to get some momentum going for the next one. It is easier to keep it going than to start and stop in the manner of yo-yo dieting.

Additionally, overnight changes are not healthy for the diet. Learning to adapt to increased fiber intake from whole grains or more vegetables takes some time for the body. Many people find that changes that occur too quickly generally lead to an overall feeling of sluggishness, fatigue and other related problems during the first few weeks, as the body adjusts and purges itself of some of the toxins that have been built up over the years. While this is necessarily unhealthy, it can be a deterrent to further change and is often frustrating to deal with. One common example of this is the caffeine headache so commonly associated with "cold turkey" quitting. Additionally, changes to real foods often result in weight loss, something that should also happen gradually to prevent many serious health concerns as the body changes too quickly. The best way to avoid these risks and concerns is to make changes slowly and gradually, allowing the body to adapt fully before moving on.

Set Attainable Goals

Even with the one step at a time approach, if the first step is to cut out the family's favorite dish, replacing it with something dramatically different, the challenge may prove to be too much. Likewise, if you allow yourself just one week to meet a new goal before moving on to the next, you could be setting yourself up for failure. Instead, be realistic with the goals and deadlines you give yourself and your family.

Setting attainable goals is the best way to ensure the plan is workable and allows the maximum opportunity to meet the goals, enjoying the benefits of a healthier diet, rather than the stress of changing too quickly. Meals should be enjoyable, not stressful and with healthy, real foods, there is no reason to make something challenging or difficult when it should be fun and inviting.

Slow and Steady Wins the Race

I have found that the best way to meet each goal is to work gradually. Instead of dumping the bleached white bread and baking a batch of whole wheat sourdough bread, which most families immediately reject, a gradual introduction to the nutty, tangy flavor of whole wheat sourdough can be slowly increased until they find they actually prefer the taste.

For flour, try substituting 10% of the white flour with whole wheat. Chances are, nobody will even notice. Stick with this for a few days, and then increase it to 20%. A few days later, try 30%, then 40% then half. Gradually, the whole-wheat flour will completely replace the white flour; meanwhile the family has had the time to adjust to the difference in taste. When this happens, they will suddenly notice that a slice of bread baked with refined, white flour has a gummy, bland taste, and lifelong habits will have been established.

For breads, baking at home may be too much of a task to begin with, and if that is the case, consider looking for a local bakery that bakes real bread. I always ask to see the ingredient list and look for the word "yeast." If it is not there, they use a natural starter, and the bread is going to be so much better than most (sometimes all) of what is available at a grocery store.

Most healthy eating habits lend themselves well to baby steps. If the children love sodas, start changing to organic sodas, moving to fruit juice based carbonated drinks, then to homemade fizzy juice drinks from Chapter Ten for parties and special celebrations.

Quality Over Quantity

Another benefit to the slow and steady approach is that it allows time to focus on quality, not quantity. Anyone can spend a fortune purchasing new ingredients and home appliances and start baking whole-wheat snacks, homemade breads and real foods tomorrow, but without the benefit of experience, the results will be less than stellar. Learning how to prepare grass fed meats takes some time, as they cook differently than conventional meats. Whole grains don't work in every recipe and many additional minor changes will need to be made.

By mastering each skill before moving on, the quality of your homemade goods will be unbeatable. Any home cook can verify that the first homemade loaf of bread was great, but nothing like the 50th. As each loaf is prepared, the baker learns how the dough should feel, how weather affects the dough, how to tweak things a touch to perfect the recipe and how to bake it just the right way. The same is true for using new flours, new kitchen tools, new types of meat and new oils and fats.

Real foods are not only superior nutritionally, but also in taste and sustainability. Unfortunately, many well-intended health food junkies have introduced some sub par products, leading many to believe that healthy foods are the opposite of delicious foods! The reality is that everything that makes a food healthy also makes it delicious. Gourmet chefs will be the first to choose real oils and fats over hydrogenated counterfeits. Processed foods were not introduced to the market for their superior taste and flavor, but as a way to cut corners, which they have done in price, taste, and appearance.

Become a Foodie

This focus on quality has led many health food enthusiasts to become fans of gourmet cooking, otherwise known as *foodies*. Foodies love to explore delicious tastes and prepare lavish meals for fun. Being a foodie does not have to be expensive; it just means you like to enjoy your food, which many health professionals recommend for proper digestion and better health. Sitting around a relaxed meal allows the body to take a break and allows the food to be properly digested, preventing many intestinal concerns, which are so common today.

Learning how to best prepare fresh foods is another trademark of the foodie, and this new hobby is a great way to make real foods fun and enjoyable. The best foods are made with only a few ingredients, but the best quality available. Instead of masking the natural flavors with harsh additives, these gourmet foods are prepared with simple, seasonal, local high quality ingredients, which bring their own intense flavors to the table.

What to Eat, Not What Not to Eat

Enjoying your food also means focusing on what *to* eat, not what not to eat - as is so common among those who stick to rigid rules and guidelines. Eating is a requirement for life, but one to be enjoyed and savored, not rushed and filled with rules. By focusing on what not to eat, mealtimes become both drudgery and a chore.

Instead of focusing on lists of ingredients to avoid, focus on foods to enjoy. Look for whole foods that can be prepared with minimal ingredients and will suit your family's diet and tastes. Use some of the recipes in this book or another whole foods book for starting points and focus on those high quality ingredients. The simple action of changing the mindset from a *don't* to a *do* makes a world of difference.

The same is true for children and for close friends and family members. When grandparents are watching the kids, leaving them with a list of what not to eat generally leaves the grandparents few choices, but leaving foods brought from home or a list of foods on hand that are suitable and that your children enjoy makes the change much more enjoyable for everyone.

Expect Setbacks

Regardless of determination and commitment, setbacks do occur. Anticipate them and work around them instead of letting them become discouraging. As new food guidelines are being established, roadblocks will arise in the form of dinner out at a favorite traditional location, meals or gatherings over at friends' houses, and even school parties, sporting events or theme parks. When children are involved, they may not understand why the traditions are being changed, and friends may not understand why your tastes have changed. Blending the need to be a graceful hostess and guest with meeting your family's nutritional goals is always a difficult and time-consuming task.

These social reasons are yet another great argument for the slow and steady approach, and when things occur that don't fit the plan, don't let it become discouraging. Instead, simply modify the plan, change a few deadlines or goals, and move forward again. Even the best-laid plans will run into some unexpected occurrences, and even the healthiest families have to take unanticipated shortcuts from time to time. As the family adjusts to real foods, these short cuts will become fewer and fewer, and progress will continue to be made. As with anything, they are an unavoidable part of the process.

Where to Begin?

The next step is to set some goals and make a plan! I've included some ideas as a jumping off point, but it is important to carefully analyze each goal, making sure it is suitable for your family's unique dietary and health needs. Modify and adjust them as needed to make them your own, or come up with your own personal goals to meet! Generally, six to eight weeks is a good time frame to meet one of the goals set below, but if the change is a big one, it may take much more time to implement.

These goals are grouped by topic, so if some of them are already a part of your family's routine, you can look to the next step beneath it for a more advanced option. I recommend adding your own goals and adjusting these to suit your family's health and tastes, and then prioritizing them. Once this is done, start with the first goal and work your way through. Some more difficult tasks may need a year or two to implement, and others may require new skills or kitchen appliances that need to be worked into the budget, so keep those things in mind as you plan.

- Begin adding whole-wheat flour to baked goods, gradually eliminating white or refined flours.
- Eliminate sodas.
- Add three to four servings of fruits and vegetables to the diet daily.
- Increase that number to five to seven.
- Join a CSA (Community Supported Agriculture).
- Find other sources of local, organic or naturally grown foods and produce.
- Plant a kitchen herb garden.
- Plant a vegetable garden.
- Plant a berry bush or fruit / nut tree.
- Begin eliminating hydrogenated oils from the diet.
- Begin eliminating high fructose corn syrup,
- Begin using natural sweetening options, eliminating refined sugars.
- Reduce animal meats to three to five servings per week.
- Change to free range, grass fed, antibiotic and hormone free meats.
- Look for local providers of animal meats, dairy and eggs.
- Start packing snacks or a lunch to avoid fast food.
- Begin baking bread or making fresh cheese at home.
- Learn new ways to prepare foods without refined or processed ingredients.
- Locate and experience restaurants that serve meals made with fresh, organic and / or local ingredients.
- Add your family's goals here:

Chapter Ten: Real Foods for Real Kids

While children may benefit the most from a household change to real foods, if they have been consuming the traditional childhood fare, the change may meet some resistance, especially at first. Of course, this doesn't have to be determined by a battle of wills, and shouldn't be reduced to strict parenting methods. Bringing kids on board with healthy meal options can be surprisingly easy - even with the pickiest of eaters. The key is to find your creative side and make the new foods just as fun as the processed products. Don't feel like you have a creative side in the kitchen? The recipes and ideas at the end of this chapter will help with that!

Despite initial hindrances, some of the most dedicated healthy eaters I've met are children. They like their world to make sense, and though they enjoy bright colors and playful characters on the food, they also like knowing that the food they eat will benefit them. Once children, especially younger children, learn the benefits of healthy foods, and adapt to the flavors and textures, they often are the first to object when compromises are made - and the most willing to turn down processed foods.

However, if they don't know that milk comes from a cow and that strawberries grow in the ground, and the only foods they've experienced are processed, molded into shapes and colored and flavored to match their favorite cartoon character, the first step is to get them to enjoy a diet of real foods.

Reasonable Expectations

If the majority of their foods are colored, shaped and flavored, they will probably immediately reject the whole grain natural flavors that are new and different. This is not, as commonly believed, because children don't like healthy foods. It is because children, in general, like predictability and don't like changes. Whole grain bread feels different in the mouth. It looks different on the plate and the peanut butter and jelly are not quickly absorbed, resulting in changes from their expectations. Their palates are no less suited to enjoy the foods than an adult's; they just prefer to remain with what they are comfortable looking at, feeling and tasting.

Therefore, to change their habits doesn't mean the bread needs to look or feel like their old bread, though that could be beneficial during the transition period. More importantly, they simply need the time to adjust to these new changes, and the repeated exposure that enables these foods to become familiar, thus comfortable. After all, most child-friendly foods are known to adults as comfort food.

To help with this, set reasonable expectations. Instead of serving the new foods and insisting they learn to love them, remember that it often takes many, many exposures to a food for a child to learn whether or not they like it. When introducing a new food to my own children, I often give them only one bean, or an equally small portion of the new item. They eat just the little bite or two in addition to the rest of the meal, which is already familiar to them. After ensuring that this new food has been seen on the plate once or twice a week for a month or more, I usually find that one of them begins requesting it, and their portion size grows as they learn they enjoy it. Of course, there are the occasions when a child simply does not prefer that flavor, which is a different situation entirely.

Think Outside of the Box (or Schedule)

Another characteristic children are known for is to ignore traditional menus. They don't always feel like breakfast foods in the morning or dinner foods at night, and their idea of a well-rounded meal may vary from an adult's. Instead of worrying about the appearance of their plates, I worry about the foods that are on them.

In practical terms, my children may have chips with "bean dip" for lunch. As long as the chips are organic, natural corn chips (or homemade chips) and the bean dip is a recipe I've made from healthy beans and spices, the end result is not much different than a bean burrito, but the presentation and layout is different. If they will eat more real foods when the ingredients are presented one way, I don't worry too much about making it fit my pre-conceived notions of what a healthy plate looks like!

Likewise, while traveling, I've often fed my children crackers for breakfast with fresh fruits, hummus and some cheese. While many would balk at that admission, I have no problems with it. I would much prefer that they eat something slightly unconventional while still receiving plenty of various nutrients, than to serve them a bowl of "appropriate" breakfast cereal, which offers little more than refined sugar, artificial flavors and colors, and a bit of hydrogenated oil.

Thinking outside of the traditional menu options often appeals to little ones as exciting and adventurous. Additionally, focusing on the actual nutritional value of the food (not counting fats and calories, but aiming for a variety of fruits, vegetables and real, whole foods) instead of the traditional notions of time appropriate meals generally provides children with a much healthier overall diet.

So the next time they ask for hummus for breakfast or an egg for lunch, think about all the nutritional benefits from these whole foods, instead of what the clock says they should eat.

Little Sous-Chefs

Children are more likely to eat foods that they have helped to prepare. Knowing what went into the item provides some security that the item is actually good and encourages them to take pride in their work.

While they do make messes, and are not quite ready for every kitchen skill, covering the basics when they are young establishes healthy eating habits that will last a lifetime. The ability to walk into a kitchen and actually prepare food is an art that is quickly fading from society, as most people now confuse heating an item for cooking, which involves actual ingredient selection, food preparation, arranging the items and typically ends with the application of heat. Unwrapping a product and setting a timer is not cooking, and emptying a box into a bowl, adding eggs and tossing into the oven is only one small step closer.

Getting children into the kitchen as little ones and enabling them to feel comfortable with fresh ingredients, watching and observing all of the steps along the way and enjoying the final result helps them to enjoy the real foods much more than if they merely sat down at the table. It also teaches them how foods are made, what to expect from food preparation, how to chop, arrange, prepare, etc., and other useful skills that are not taught by keeping them out of the kitchen.

Though it does take additional time and patience, including children in the entire process of mealtime is worth every bit of effort.

Join Them At The Table

This is a piece of advice promoted by nearly everyone, but in our busy lives is rarely actually accomplished. However, research shows that children eat healthier foods when their parents join them at the dinner table. Professionals also agree that eating foods at the table, as opposed to the couch, desk, car, or other location, results in consumption of healthier foods and establishes better lifelong habits for all involved.

One of the reasons we tend to rely on quick and processed foods is convenience, and this habit is quickly passed along to our children. Taking the time to prepare a meal and sitting down to consume the foods shows our children that food is important and the task of fueling our bodies is not one to be rushed or skimped on.

This is not only true for dinnertime; the same is true for breakfast, lunch and snack-time. Most children's snacks are sold in single serving pre-packaged containers that seldom provide any real nourishment and are a waste of valuable resources. Instead of making mealtime a last minute chore, plan ahead. Prepare snacks ahead of time that can be ready in little time, but provide nourishment. Carrots, grapes, and other raw fruits and veggies are perfect for keeping little tummies full between meals and even combo options like cheese and crackers can be prepared ahead of time and kept in the fridge until needed.

Real Foods Can Be Fun

Though children naturally learn to enjoy healthy foods, one of the main reasons they request processed foods is the simple fact that they look like fun. There is no reason real foods can't be fun! We've managed to celebrate every holiday and birthday with healthy foods for not only our families but also guests who are not accustomed to eating natural foods, and everyone has enjoyed the food. Most guests don't even realize that the foods they are enjoying are healthier, aside from the lack of processed candy in the party favors. We make allergen free cupcakes with natural sweeteners and ice them with coconut oil based frosting and herb colored sprinkles, and we rarely have leftovers. We make homemade pizza dough and let the kids top them as they like; we make homemade lemonade and anything else a party or holiday should have. They don't miss out on any of the fun, but they do safely avoid hydrogenated oils, high fructose corn syrup, artificial colors and flavors, excessive sugars and any other ingredients that have the ability to lower their immune system and adversely affect their development. Even Easter eggs can be naturally dyed with herbs and plants for fun, colorful eggs without the worry.

Recipe, Tips and Suggestions:

I've included some of my favorite recipes below. These have been successfully used in my home with my four children, and make great starting points for a healthier (yet kid-friendly) diet. Once you begin cooking with real, natural ingredients, you will find that you can still use your favorite cookbooks. Just tweak with the ingredient list by substituting healthier ingredients for those that are not suitable for children. Sometimes a little trial and error is necessary, but the results are always worth it!

Chicken Nuggets, Gluten Free

The gluten free diet has shown to be life changing for some children, primarily those with digestive or developmental challenges such as celiac, ADHD or autism. Yet, despite the great success many parents enjoy from the diet, it is one of the most difficult lifestyle changes to undertake as gluten is in many, many products. Sometimes it is the little things that make a huge difference for children on a gluten free diet. While chicken nuggets may not be widely recognized as a health food, they are a staple in most children's diets. These nuggets are not only gluten free, they are additive free, making them much healthier than any drive through can offer!

2 boneless, skinless chicken breasts
1/2 cup polenta
1/2 cup cornmeal
1 medium egg, beaten

dash salt and pepper
1 t Italian blend herbs

Cut the breasts into small cubes. Set aside. In a bowl, combine the grains and seasoning. Drop the nuggets into the bowl and coat lightly. Next, dredge the nuggets through the beaten egg until moistened well. Place them again into the dry mixture, taking care to coat the nuggets thoroughly.

Place the nuggets onto a lightly greased baking sheet. Bake at 400 degrees for 20-25 minutes. Serve hot with plenty of gluten free dipping sauces. (As an alternative, the nuggets can be fried in medium hot oil until golden brown and crispy.)

Coconut Candy

This is one of my favorite candy recipes. Not only is it extremely low in sugar, it offers a powerful nutritional contribution to the diet, and is great for failure to thrive children or those of any age that can use some healthy fats, but have a picky palate.

Take about 1/2 cup of coconut oil and mix in 2 T blue agave and 2 T raw honey. Once thoroughly combined, add 1 and a half cups of grated coconut. Then, with a small cookie scoop, measure out little balls, carefully shaping them before the oil melts then place in the fridge to cool. Once chilled, dip into melted chocolate chips (the dairy free, real cocoa butter and real vanilla kind.) When the chocolate begins to set, top with a little flake of coconut and place back in the fridge to harden.

The candies boast a whopping 10-14 g of healthy raw coconut oil fat, very little sugar (so little to no spike in blood sugar levels) and assorted trace nutrients. Even more impressive is the utter lack of hydrogenated oils, refined sugars and common allergens such as gluten and nuts! It can easily be made raw (sub raw cocoa nibs for chocolate and mix into the filing instead of dipping) or vegan (use all agave instead of honey) Not bad for a *treat*!

Electrolyte drinks are a staple in the home with a pregnant mother or small child. They help prevent dehydration during labor and childhood illnesses. Yet, the ingredient list is often pretty scary. If you have never looked at one, you would probably be appalled at what you see. They are not at all natural, and certainly nothing we want to give a sick baby or child (or laboring mama). However, dehydration is a real concern and the concept of an electrolyte drink is a good one indeed, which is why we like to make these all natural drinks at home. (Tip: Be sure to use mineral salt and pure, natural ingredients!)

Lemon-aide
1 cup water
1 T lemon juice
1/4 t salt
pinch baking soda
1 T honey

Cran-aide
1 cup water
1/3 cup cranberry juice
1/4 t salt
pinch baking soda

Other Flavors
1 cup water
1/3 cup grape juice / orange juice / berry juice
1/4 t salt
pinch baking soda

Fizzy Drinks: These are such fun treats for little ones, but the conventional varieties are typically packed with unhealthy ingredients. Instead, these natural drinks offer trace minerals and assorted vitamins. Their sugars are purely natural and their taste is far superior! Simply blend 1 can of (thawed) juice concentrate with 1 liter of carbonated water. Stir gently, to avoid allowing the drink to become "flat" and serve over ice.

Fruit Punch: Fruit punch is another staple in many homes with little ones, but the store bought version is typically nothing but high fructose corn syrup, artificial colors and flavors, and perhaps a little real juice thrown in for good measure. At the next birthday party or play group, try this natural version instead - not only is it healthier than the corn syrup concoctions, the flavor is unbeatable! (Note: This is still a sweet beverage and in a healthy home it would be reserved for special occasions!) Take 1 can of each organic frozen juice concentrate: cranberry, orange, lemonade and grape. Blend together with the recommended amount of water in a large container. Serve chilled.

Ice Cream Sandwiches, Gluten Free

My motto is that no real food is bad, they have just been prepared with terrible recipes. Many favorite junk foods could actually be a great part of a real foods diet, as long as they are prepared correctly and kept in moderation. Ice cream and ice cream sandwiches are a great example of this. Any natural chocolate cookie can be used for a traditional sandwich. Below is a gluten free option for children that do not need to consume gluten. These ice cream sandwiches so good that even guests who are not on a gluten-free diet will love them!

1/2 cup brown rice flour
1/4 cup cornstarch
1 T garbanzo bean flour
1/4 cup cocoa powder
1 stick butter
1/4 cup chocolate chips
1 cup sucanat
1/4 cup agave nectar
1 t salt
3 eggs
2 t vanilla extract

Over low heat, melt the butter and chocolate chips together. Remove from heat and add the sugar, salt, eggs and vanilla. When combined, add the remaining dry ingredients. The mixture will resemble brownie batter. Spread in a thin layer onto a lined cookie sheet. Bake at 350 for 12-15 minutes or until a toothpick comes clean. While still warm, pierce with a fork and score into squares (or cut into circles using a ice cream sandwich mold). When cooled, pack a scoop of softened ice cream in between 2 cookies and place in the freezer to firm. Makes 6-12 sandwiches, depending on size of squares.

Lunchbox Sandwiches are also staples in the home with little ones. They are simple to toss together, can be adjusted to any dietary preferences (i.e. vegetarian, allergen free, etc) and are easily portable. Yet, the same old peanut butter and jelly can become boring quickly, and leaves plenty of room for improvement nutritionally. Here are some classic combinations that help liven things up a bit:

- Apple Swiss (apple slices with Swiss cheese)
- Sunflower Butter and Honey (just about 1 T of honey)
- Strawberry Jam and Cream Cheese (organic of course!)
- Almond Butter and Apples (slice thin for best results)
- Turkey and Cream Cheese (for older palates, add a touch of dried herbs)
- Sunflower Butter, Raisins and Celery
- Cinnamon Cream Cheese (to 8oz cream cheese, add 1 T honey and 1 t cinnamon)
- Cashew Butter and Sliced Bananas
- California Veggie (cream cheese, sun dried tomatoes and avocado slices)
- Turkey and Green Apple with Cream Cheese
- Fruit Salad (cream cheese spread on bread with sliced apples and bananas)

Natural Egg Dyes

These are fun and easy to make, requiring just a little additional time collecting the materials, and they result in beautiful, natural hues that liven up any spring table.

vinegar
distilled water
herbs for colors (see below for a guide)
boiled eggs

For each color, mix 4 cups of water with 4 T of the herb powder or 3/4 cup of the whole herb and 3T vinegar. Bring to a boil and boil for 20 -25 minutes. Strain and cool. Soak eggs for 10 -15 minutes in the dye. Dry in egg cups, then store in the fridge.

Color Guide:
Blue - red cabbage or blueberry concentrate
Brown - ground tea or coffee

Burnt Orange - red chili powder
Green - spinach powder or parsley powder
Red - cranberries
Orange - curry powder
Pink - beet powder
Purple - beets, purple onion skin, grape juice
Yellow - calendula petals, turmeric or saffron

Polka Dot Cookies

Cookies are always a great way to sneak in some additional whole grains and nutrients. They are small, portable, easy to bake, and extremely kid-friendly. These polka dot cookies help children learn to love quinoa, a versatile and healthy grain. Any type of quinoa can be used. Red gives the cookies a more colorful appearance that is often a hit, but black is also very fun. If you cook the quinoa for dinner and save a bit before adding savory herbs, this can be made the following day with the reserved quinoa, saving even more time.

1 1/2 cups whole wheat flour
2 eggs
1/2 cup sucanat
1/2 cup honey
2 t vanilla extract
1 t cinnamon
1 cup quinoa, cooked
2/3 cup oats
1/2 cup organic butter
2 t baking powder
1 t salt

Combine the sweeteners and butter in a bowl and blend well. Add eggs, one at a time, then add the vanilla. Combine the flour, cinnamon, salt and baking powder and add that mixture to the wet ingredients. Gently stir in the oats and quinoa. Scoop into 1-2 T portions and bake on an ungreased cookie sheet in a preheated 350 degree oven for 12-15 minutes or until golden brown. For additional polka dots, try adding 1/2 cup of dried cranberries or golden raisins.

Tri Color Orzo

Orzo is nothing more than small, rice shaped pasta. The colors come from vegetable extracts, making it naturally kid friendly and healthy! This dish is a standby in our home. It needs to spend some time in the fridge for the flavors to blend, which makes it a perfect make ahead dish for busy evenings. It is best served chilled, but can also be served at room temperature and can be prepared up to 2 days in advance! For picky eaters, feel free to substitute any of the ingredients for those that are more familiar and comfortable.

1 pound tri color orzo
1/4 cup sun dried tomatoes, drained
1/2 cup Kalamata olives
8-10 artichoke hearts, drained
1/2 cup Italian herbed vinaigrette
1/4 cup shredded hard Italian cheese such as Parmesan
2-3 T pine nuts

Cook pasta according to package directions. (Do not overcook!) Rinse well with cool water. Stir in the vinaigrette, olives, tomatoes and artichokes. Chill, covered, for 2-4 hours. Remove and top with the cheese and nuts before serving.

Chapter Eleven: Real Foods on a Budget

Perhaps with the exception of picky eaters in the house (usually children, as we've discussed), the most common concern I hear from parents who want to change to real foods is that the cost is prohibitive. This is usually a fair argument, considering that most unhealthy and processed foods have been artificially cheapened, thanks in part to subsidies. If the diet looks the same but organic and local ingredients are substituted for the processed and conventional foods, the price will dramatically increase.

But to take the pantry, empty it, then replace everything with the organic version is not to change to a real foods diet. It may be healthier, but it would be missing the point entirely. And the real health benefits, interestingly enough, come from the most sustainable foods, which probably don't look like the foods currently in your pantry or fridge.

In my experience, having helped numerous families transition to diets of real foods, it does not have to cost more. Many families actually discover that their grocery budget with real foods is lower than when they were buying conventional foods. However, these results require more than a change in the grocery list. They are a lifestyle change, which is the collective result of reversing many old habits and establishing many new ones. That process does not happen overnight, and it does not necessarily result in immediate budgetary savings.

That being said, the argument that real foods are too expensive is one to address head on, even if it is possible to consume real foods on a smaller budget. Michael Pollan, author of *The Omnivore's Dilemma*, has said, "The less we spend on food, the more we spend on healthcare." Purchasing cheap foods at the grocery store may seem to be the answer to a salary cut or a failing economy, but this type of living is not much different than living on a credit card. The deal seems great now, but the real cost is coming - and will be much more than we bargained for.

As we discussed in the first section, these foods come at a cost to our health. These health concerns not only result in decreased immunity, but real, life-long problems, many of which impact the health of our offspring for the next two or three generations! An entirely new field of science known as epigenetics evaluates these health concerns and their impact on our children's children. For the first time in two centuries, America's children are expected to experience a shorter life expectancy than their parents. These are serious consequences that extend far beyond our pocketbooks.

In addition to the impact our food choices make on future generations, many of the compounded costs of poor quality foods will directly affect our own bank accounts, resulting in immediate loss of any savings at the grocery store. When families consume foods that lead to decreased immunity, they lose days of work, often without pay; they spend more on medicine, doctors' visits, childcare, and other related costs. Health insurance costs skyrocket, doctors' visits and pharmacy costs increase, working days decrease and productivity is reduced. Suddenly the $50 saved at the grocery store doesn't seem like such a bargain after all.

Our reactive system of healthcare is expensive and time consuming. Sure, it may cost an additional $2 for a different type of milk, but when it prevents recurring ear infections, which are often linked to dairy sensitivities, the savings includes the doctor's co pay, the prescription cost and, in many cases, the cost of more intense treatments when the antibiotic doesn't clear it up - which professionals have been telling us for over a decade.

Wellness does cost money - either through providing nourishing and healthy foods for our families, or through paying for the countless office visits, prescriptions and days lost from work for the illness and diseases that have been linked to the standard diet. Diabetes, obesity and infertility have been called epidemic, and the cost to treat these conditions has reached tens of billions of dollars. Eczema, allergies and gastrointestinal problems have become the norm, and ear infections or tubes are standard fare for childhood. What if proper nutrition and prevention methods could prevent the majority of these cases? According to research, that is feasible.

Therefore, the real question might be: Can we afford not to eat healthy? Can we afford to increase our chances of the overwhelming number of diseases that have been directly linked to poor diet?

Real Cost of Healthier Diets

Fortunately, the actual cost of real foods has been grossly exaggerated. By changing lifestyles and habits, real foods can be obtained without breaking the budget, but it takes some determination and willingness to change.

In fact, families that don't have budgetary constraints often have more trouble adapting a real foods diet because they *do* have the option of merely purchasing organic versions of conventional foods. In other words, their eating habits and food choices are not changing; they are merely eliminating pesticides and GMOs (genetically modified organisms). Those are important steps, but they only scratch the surface. Many processed organic foods are available at health food stores nationwide.

These tips are not listed in any particular order. Some may work for your family while others don't, and that is fine. Read over them, find what works, and include those in your plan for a healthier diet. Or select certain aspects of each tip and work your way through them slowly - whatever works best for you. You may find that once you begin eating healthier foods, making the time for your diet is not the drudgery you once believed it to be.

Rethinking the Grocery List

One of the best ways to add healthier foods on a tight budget is to change your grocery list. Take the old one and throw it away. Actually, hold on to it long enough to use it as a reference for a new one - then toss it. Remove anything that is ready to serve or ready to bake. Cooking involves more than just heating, and these foods are, essentially, instant food - never a good option. Instead, think about the ingredients used to prepare these dishes and add those to your new list. Instead of refrigerated cookie dough, add natural chocolate chips, flour (or grain if you grind your own) and butter to the list. Instead of frozen lasagna, add lasagna noodles, tomato sauce (or tomatoes) and some cheese to the list.

Frozen pizza can be replaced with flour, tomato sauce and cheese as well - so you can buy larger amounts of those ingredients, saving even more! Items to omit from the list: most frozen foods, snack sized packages of foods, everything on the cookie / cracker aisle, anything ready to bake or ready to serve, and most items with more than 6-8 ingredients on the label.

Some of the more expensive items left on your list may be the meat, oil, dairy products and herbs / spices. Natural sugar alternatives can also be expansive when compared to white sugar. This natural pricing actually serves as a good reminder of the correct balance these items should represent in our diets. Most of us are buying far too much meat, sugar and dairy, and healthy diets generally recommend a reduction in each of those key areas. Limiting that intake to organic, healthy versions also helps to maintain the natural ratio of foods in the diet. When sugar and butter are not available in abundance, snacking habits change, recipes are altered and overall health improves! (As a side note - these items are also some of the most important items to purchase in organic form. Toxins accumulate in the fat of mammals, so dairy products, especially butter and cheese, will also contain more of these unwanted substances.)

Don't panic if your list grows. It will. However, each new item will cost a fraction of the prepackaged food you're accustomed to buying, so the overall total will not jump that much. Pre-packaged foods typically cost 2-3 times as much as the raw ingredients, despite the inferior ingredient list. Buying ingredients also allows you to buy some items in bulk, increasing the saving potential.

Do It Yourself (DIY)

So, now that the pantry is packed with actual ingredients, not foods that have already been prepared, the next step is to make foods at home from scratch. This is the perfect way to know everything that goes into your food, ensuring fresh and high quality ingredients, and eliminating any need for preservatives or other additives. This increases the quality and flavor of the foods the family consumes.

While the DIY in the kitchen concept is hardly new, it is typically applied to the same foods - lasagna, casseroles, stir-fry, chicken nuggets, and so on. These are all great foods to prepare at home, and by working on double or triple sized batches, you can create your own quick frozen meals. However, the DIY benefits in the kitchen shouldn't end there.

Everything on the sauce / condiment aisle can be prepared at home for a mere fraction of the cost. Salad dressings, especially vinaigrettes, marinades, sauces and even garnishments are grossly overpriced and even the organic, natural versions contain various preservatives, stabilizers, thickeners, emulsifiers and other assorted additives. The truth is, it is not at all complicated to create your own. It is simple, requires very few ingredients, no special equipment and can be completed in minutes. I like to store the vinaigrettes and other sauces in a (labeled) glass canning jar. This inexpensive option is easy to clean, uniform in size (so the lids are interchangeable), and I can just grab the jar, shake it use it, and then toss it into the dishwasher. Simple as can be.

Cookies, desserts and baked goods are other simple items that can be made home for a fraction of the price in a short amount of time, and the final product far exceeds the store bought version in quality and flavor. It's a win-win for everyone.

At the Grocer

The big box style grocery store, despite first appearances, is one of the toughest places to save money on real foods, but with a little creativity, real foods can still be found at reasonable prices. Some of these new habits may seem daunting at first, but are typically quite simple to adapt and usually end up being fairly fun as well.

Sticking with ingredients, not pre-packaged foods, is the best way to cut costs at a grocery store. Dried grains, frozen organic fruits, dairy products and some dried herbs / seasonings are the best items to look for here. Fresh produce, fresh herbs, meats and other items are best grown at home or purchased through local resources. For larger families, grains and seasonings can be obtained in larger quantities through natural food co-ops.

Buying these ingredients in larger sizes will often dramatically reduce the total cost of the grocery bill. Cheeses, frozen fruits and vegetables, and grains all lend themselves well to bulk storage, and are commonly used in many recipes, so they don't last long at home.

As for the fruits and vegetables - it may seem odd to purchase frozen varieties, but if the item is out of season locally, the only "fresh" produce available will have been shipped from far away, is less likely to be organic, and due to these factors, will be quite nutrient poor. Frozen fruits and vegetables, however, are typically harvested ripe, frozen within a short period of time and naturally preserved until they reach your kitchen. This results in more nutrient dense food.

Instead of the Grocer

While the grocery store may be where most people purchase the vast majority of food, it is not the ideal place to find healthy, real foods. Breaking free of this habit may be one of the healthiest and most cost effective steps you take. Local CSAs, co-ops, farmers and markets often provide better options at literally a fraction of the cost. However, flexibility may be the key here.

For example, I purchase all of my meats from a farm about ten miles away from my house. Our farmers have a completely sustainable farm with plenty of room for the animals to roam safely. The animals all consume the foods they were designed to consume and are provided safe areas to grow healthy. I can take my children to the farm anytime I want to personally see how the animals are cared for, and we are updated with all farm news - such as the birth of a new baby calf - on a regular basis. Because we buy directly from the farmers, the cost we pay for local, organic, hormone and antibiotic free food is comparable to conventional meat on sale in a traditional grocer. The benefits, however, are priceless.

Backyard or even indoor gardens are also great ways to obtain fresh, local produce for much less than the conventional options at a grocery store. Many foods are simple to grow and don't require lots of land, time or talent. Blueberry bushes and other larger plants are relatively easy to maintain, providing an annual harvest for relatively little work. Vegetable gardens may take more time, but the savings are substantial. If you don't have a large yard or the time to grow large amounts of food, you can still enjoy savings by growing your own food with a kitchen herb garden.

Even if you have never grown a plant, you can easily grow fresh culinary herbs such as basil or chives in the kitchen. Fresh organic herbs at the grocery store are extremely expensive and don't last long. Once a basil plant is established, it will grow in a pot in the kitchen, providing free fresh organic herbs whenever they are needed. Many herbal plants are native to the Mediterranean region, which means they enjoy warm, dry weather and don't need frequent watering - preferences that make growing relatively simple! This new habit not only saves quite a bit on the grocery bill; it also encourages the use of more fresh herbs in the diet. Since they are sitting right there, why not toss a few into the next dish? Herbs are concentrated sources of nutrients, particularly vitamins, minerals and antioxidants. Adding a little natural flavor to the diet can improve both your cooking skills and your family's health.

Farmers

For those who don't have a green thumb or consume more produce than can reasonably be grown at home, getting to know the local farmers is a must. Not only do most farmers sell their produce at local farmer's markets, they offer many alternative ways of obtaining produce - usually at substantial cost savings.

One such way is a CSA. Community Supported Agriculture (CSA) is a concept that benefits both local farmers and families. With this option, you agree to purchase a regular amount of produce from a local farmer on a weekly / biweekly / monthly basis when signing up or joining. The agreement usually lasts one year; then it can be renewed the following year - or not. The agreement entitles each member to one "share" of the produce, which is usually a bushel, half bushel or even a quarter bushel.

The food in the share will vary based upon what is in season currently, and the yield from that farm that year. In other words, the produce will always reflect what can be picked locally that week, and if the farmer has a bumper crop, the members get a packed box. If fewer items are ready for harvest, the box may be less full. Most good farmers prepare ahead of time to provide full boxes throughout the year by planting crops with a variety of harvesting estimates.

The box will always have whatever is in season, so members will have many opportunities to try new or unfamiliar foods. Some farmers will even allow substitutions for foods your family does not eat. In return for this agreement, the farmer provides the share at a cost that is substantially lower than the grocery store can provide. Many farmers are certified organic, but even if not, local produce is always healthier than what has traveled across the country to reach the table. CSAs often fill up early in the year - especially if they are well-established and reliable farmers! I usually register for my produce CSA in January or early February!

Local pick-your-own farms are also great ways to obtain local produce at great prices, if you're willing to do a little bit of work. These farms grow the fruit or vegetables, then allow others to come in and harvest the produce, paying a reduced rate for the items. The per pound price of the fresh produce is much less than conventional produce at a grocery store, and the pick your own farms always offer local produce, and usually provide organic or limited pesticide use items. My children and I have an annual summer tradition at a local blueberry patch. We spend about 4-5 hours early one summer morning (before it gets too hot) and all of my children fill their baskets with berries. Then we sit on the grass, enjoy a picnic and read some fun children's books about blueberries. We head home, clean up and enjoy blueberry buckle, jam and pies for the following week. Then I freeze the remaining berries and we have plenty for smoothies and desserts year round. We bring home between 10 and 15 pounds for about the cost of 2-3 pints at the grocery store. This is also a great way to teach children where real food comes from, how much work is involved with food preparation (even if it is fun work) and the difference found in fresh foods. If you've never tasted a blueberry or strawberry fresh from the plant or bush, you're in for a real treat!

Co-ops

Another great option for obtaining whole foods at reduced prices is to join a natural foods co-op. In a coop, a group of like minded individuals put their orders together to buy directly from the supplier, obtaining wholesale or near wholesale prices. Typically, co-ops have large minimums, so this would be a once a year type purchase, but items like organic ground sugarcane, flour and other grains can be bought in bulk at amazing prices. I even buy my name brand organic personal care products, dish soap, and other non-food dry goods from one of my coops - at nearly 40% off retail prices! This option requires a good deal of planning - I typically buy enough automatic dish soap to last 3-4 months - but the savings are worth it.

Some of my favorite co-ops include Something Better Natural Foods, Frontier Wholesale, Bread Beckers, and Country Life Natural Foods, but there are dozens of really great options.

A Step Further

Most of the options so far only require some careful planning, and not too much talent, but with some basic kitchen skills, the options for fresh real foods at amazing prices can be greatly expanded. Learning to bake bread or make cheese may seem like an all day task reminiscent of the pioneer days, but with modern conveniences, these projects are easy to incorporate into a healthy home.

Bread baking with a natural starter takes very little hands on time in the kitchen - just some additional planning and a little practice. Freshly grinding wheat for the bread is another seemingly daunting task that really requires nothing more than a tabletop grain mill and about five minutes. Many amazing cookbooks exist to cover the topic. I've had great success doing it the old fashioned way. After getting my starter or "mother" established, I just toss it into the next batch of dough in place of the packet of baker's yeast. Then, before adding any flavorings or other ingredients, I reserve some for next time. This allows me to use any bread recipe I find and the only modification I make is to extend the rising time by about an hour.

Cheese-making is another great way to get fresh, high quality foods for much less and it is a very kid-friendly project as well. While organic and local milk is readily available, organic cheeses are often quite expensive and difficult to find. Both ricotta and cream cheese are simple for beginners and with a few additional tools, mozzarella and other soft cheeses can be added to the repertoire of the more advanced home cheese-maker.

Homemade Ricotta requires one gallon of non-homogenized whole milk. If that is not available, take a gallon of regular organic milk and replace 1 cup of it with 1 cup of heavy cream. In addition, you will need 1/4 cup raw apple cider vinegar and 1 teaspoon sea salt. In a large saucepan, heat the milk until just before it begins to boil, about 185 degrees. Remove from heat and add the vinegar, stirring gently until the curds begin to form. When this happens, add the salt, cover with a thin cloth and leave to curdle for about 3 hours. Drain the ricotta using a sheet of cheesecloth placed over a colander. Don't dump the fresh cheese directly into the cheesecloth, gently allow them to tumble in. The cheese does not completely drain, as a bit of moisture is desirable, so once most of the liquid has been removed, transfer the cheese to a bowl. This should take about 45 minutes to an hour. Cover the bowl and store in the refrigerator up to five days.

Homemade Cream Cheese begins with 2 cups of heavy cream. Most cheese making requires the use of bacteria, but pasteurization kills all of the bacteria, so it has to be added back into the mixture. One easy way to do this is to use cultured buttermilk. This is a special kind of buttermilk, not the regular store bought kind, and it contains beneficial bacteria. If you can't find the cultured buttermilk, a real yogurt (with beneficial bacteria) will work just as well. Allow the cream to reach room temperature. A saucepan placed over very low heat will do this, but make sure it does not get above the upper 70's. Add the buttermilk or yogurt, cover the bowl, and place in a somewhat warm place about eight hours or overnight. If you make homemade bread, the location you've found for allowing the bread to rise would be perfect. When it has set, the curds should be fairly thick, not as fluffy as the ricotta curds, but recognizable. Line a colander with a sheet of cheesecloth and gently scoop the curds in, allowing them to drain. This cheese will need to drain for about 1-2 hours. Transfer to a covered bowl and store in the refrigerator up to five days.

Other Recipes and Techniques:

Basic Vinaigrette: This basic recipe is a great baseline recipe for any salad dressing. It can be updated with various oils, vinegars and additives such as cheese, nuts, dried fruits or herbs.

1/2 cup olive oil (quality is important here)
3 T raw apple cider vinegar
2 t Dijon mustard (this acts as an emulsifier, keeping the vinaigrette from separating as rapidly)
1/2 t salt
dash fresh black pepper

Beans

Cooked beans are often stored in cans that can leach chemicals and indirect additives into the food. Dried beans are a great way to avoid this and are typically much more inexpensive as well. Beans make a great, healthy protein source and are ideal for those that need a little help reducing the meat in their diets.

1 cup dried beans
3-5 cloves garlic
1-2 T olive oil
salt and pepper to taste

Place the beans in a bowl, cover with water and soak six to eight hours or overnight. Drain, rinse and place in a saucepan. Add the garlic, oil, salt, pepper and enough water to completely cover the beans by about 2 inches. bring to a boil, skim off any foam that has accumulated on the top of the water, reduce heat to low and simmer for 1-2 hours. While simmering, check the beans every 15 minutes to ensure that the water level remains 1-2 inches above the beans. The beans are ready when they are soft and tender, but not mushy. Beans can be stored in the refrigerator for 5-7 days.

Cereal Bars: On the go breakfast foods were a great idea, but most contain those dreaded words: hydrogenated oils and high fructose corn syrup. Not to mention the wastefulness of the individual wrapping and unreasonable cost. Like most of our recipes, these are simple to make at home and provide beneficial fiber and B vitamins from the whole wheat, healthy proteins and fats from the nuts, butter and grains, and just the right blend of fats/carbohydrates/proteins to jump start your day!

1 cup (2 sticks) organic butter
1/3 cup honey
1/3 cup sucanat
1 1/2 cups whole wheat flour
1/2 cup almond meal (or almond flour or ground almonds)
2 cups oats
1 cup strawberry preserves / jam
1 t vanilla extract
1/2 t salt
1/2 t baking powder

Blend the butter and sweeteners. Combine with remaining ingredients. Press 1/2 - 2/3 of the dough into a buttered square 8x8 pan. Spread the fruit on top, then press the remaining dough over the fruit. Bake at 350 degrees for 25-30 minutes. For a thinner variety (like the store bought version) use a 9x13 pan and increase the fruit to 1 1/2 cups.

Cheese Sauce

A basic cheese sauce is extremely versatile in the kitchen. It can be poured over pasta for a fast side dish or can be combined with herbs or savory seasonings for chicken, vegetables or potatoes. Most sauces contain many additives and preservatives, so mastering this kitchen essential can greatly reduce your exposure while saving quite a bit of money as well.

The type and amount of cheese will vary based on your intended use. Macaroni and cheese or another similar dish would benefit from the additional cheese, whereas potatoes or other savory dishes work better with a creamier sauce. This sauce also freezes well, so a little planning can make homemade gourmet dishes quick and easy.

2 T butter
2 T flour
2 cups milk
1-2 cups shredded cheese

Place the butter and flour in a pan over medium heat. Cook, stirring regularly, until the mixture is lightly browned and thickening. Add the milk all at once. Continue stirring with a whisk until the mixture has thickened and has a sauce-like texture. Add cheese and any additional herbs or seasonings. Combine well and use immediately or save for later use. Sauce can be frozen up to 2 months or stored in the refrigerator for 1-2 days.

Chocolate Chip Granola Bars: Granola bars have become the staple "go-to" food for traveling and long shopping trips. Yet, most granola bars are packed with hydrogenated oils, high fructose corn syrup and cheapened, artificial ingredients. These homemade treats are still sweet and dessert-like, but contain natural ingredients that our bodies recognize. The oats provide some whole grains, offsetting the sweetener content, and natural dark chocolate chips contain antioxidants! Adding walnuts or another healthy nut also contributes to the protein content and provides healthy fats that actually help our bodies lose weight! Better yet - these are simple to make and serve as a great recipe for young children learning to use the kitchen.

4 cups oats
1/2 cup dark chocolate chips (natural, with cocoa butter, not hydrogenated oils)
2/3 cup brown rice syrup (honey or a blend of agave nectar and a sugar syrup can also be used)
1/3 cup sucanat (ground sugarcane)
3 T organic butter
2 t vanilla extract (fair trade, organic)
1 t salt
1 cup chopped nuts (optional)

Preheat the oven to 350 degrees. Butter a 9x9 inch baking pan; set aside. Spread the oats and nuts over a large baking sheet and toast in preheated oven for 10-12 minutes, stirring every 2-3 minutes. Set aside to cool. In a small saucepan, mix the sweeteners together over low heat until the sucanat dissolves and the two are thoroughly blended. Set aside to cool. Once cooled, toss everything together in a large bowl, and stir to combine thoroughly. Press mixture into the prepared pan and bake for 25-30 minutes. When cooled, cut into 12 large or 16 regular sized bars.

Homemade Pizzas (dough recipe makes 12 crusts): Frozen pizzas are not only convenient, they can be a great at-home healthy "fast food" for busy days. This recipe makes 12 small sized pizza crusts - perfect for small families OR big families with a variety of palates.

12 cups whole wheat flour
3 packets baker's yeast (for naturally leavened dough, use 1 cup of sourdough starter and increase the rising time by 1 hour)
1/4 cup olive oil
1 T salt
2 T honey
6 cups water (give or take 1/2 cup, depending on the humidity)

Combine everything in a large bowl. If using a stand mixer, mix in 2 batches with the dough hook, and then hand-knead it all together. Otherwise, hand-knead the dough until it is pliable and smooth. Leave lightly covered to rise 1-2 hours or until doubled. Divide the dough into 12 equal sized balls. Let rest 10 minutes then flatten to form 8 inch discs. If using right away, glaze with olive oil and place your desired toppings.

Bake at 500 degrees for 8-10 minutes until the crust is golden brown and the cheese is bubbly. With the remaining discs, bake at 500 for 3-5 minutes until the dough is cooked but not browned. Remove and allow to cool. Freeze 2-3 hours, then wrap tightly in plastic wrap. Place back in the freezer until ready to use (up to 2-3 months) To use, remove and allow to thaw partially - about 20 minutes. Apply toppings and bake at 500 degrees until browned.

Whipped Cream

Homemade whipped cream is much healthier than the artificial stuff in a tub, and is fairly inexpensive as well. It is great on ice cream sundaes, homemade strawberry shortcake and even homemade hot cocoa on a cold morning!

1 cup heavy cream
1-2 T organic sugar or sucanat

In a medium bowl, combine the cream and sweetener, and beat with a whisk — or an electric mixer with a whisk attachment — until stiff peaks form. Store in the refrigerator for up to 3-4 hours.

Section Four: Let Your Food Be Your Medicine

Food Guide:

Hippocrates said, "**Let your food be your medicine and your medicine be your food**." There is quite a bit of wisdom in that statement, especially considering how our food intake directly affects our health. To better understand the benefits of many common foods, I've covered over 150 individual foods, including how to incorporate them into the diet.

Agar Agar

Agar agar is sometimes called the vegetarian gelatin. While commercial gelatin is made from the bones, ligaments and other parts of pigs, cows and horses, agar agar is red marine algae, which is an effective gelling agent.

Not only does it work as a natural Jell-O, it also offers numerous health benefits. The smooth mucilage soothes the digestive tract on the way down, and it also adds bulk to stools, functioning as a mild laxative.

Typically purchased as a powder or in flake form, agar agar can also be used in homemade jellies and jams and is calorie free. To make homemade jellies, add 1/2 teaspoon agar agar powder to 1 cup of liquid or mashed fruit. The mixture will not gel if it contains wine, vinegar, rhubarb or spinach, due to the acetic or oxalic acids found in those foods.

To become more familiar with agar agar, try this yummy dessert that doubles as a kid friendly laxative or soothing sore throat treatment.

Natural Gelatin

4 cups juice (apple, grape, strawberry or try a blend)
2 t agar agar powder

Combine both ingredients in a pan and cook on medium heat until boiling. Stir as it cooks for about 1 minute. Pour into a shallow pan and stick in the fridge for about 30 minutes. Cut into squares and serve in a glass cafeteria-style dish for a nostalgic snack. Or, increase the agar agar to 3 or even 4 teaspoons to make wiggly shapes with cookie cutters.

Almonds (prunus dulcis)

Arguably one of the most nutritious nuts available, almonds provide a powerful nutritional profile. These nuts come from the same family as peaches, plums and apricots, and among their boasts is the fact that they are one of the only nuts to alkalize the body.

Almonds are high in protein, a few B vitamins, iron, calcium, potassium and phosphorus. They make an ideal vegetarian protein source and they can also be made into milks and butters.

Almond butter is a great alternative to peanut butter, and is far healthier. It is also fairly easy to make at home. Simply blend raw almonds (or toasted for a distinct nutty flavor) in a blender or processor until creamy. For a smoother texture, add up to a tablespoon of flavorless oil. Want a crunchy texture? Stir in chopped almonds. This butter recipe can also be used with other nuts to make an assortment of fresh nut butters.

Be sure to save a cup of almond butter for these yummy healthy candies that pack a protein punch. These are a great treat for children who are on the smaller side and could use a little additional fat., particularly those who are picky eaters, as they easily pass for candy!

Almond Butter Crunchies

1 cup almond butter (creamy or crunchy)
1 cup oats
1 cup brown rice crisps (available from a whole foods co-op)
1/4 cup liquid sweetener
1/4 cup ground almonds
dash sea salt

1/2 t vanilla extract

For the liquid sweetener, use whatever your family prefers. This recipe works well with agave nectar, brown rice syrup, molasses or honey. Each of these sweeteners will lend a slightly different flavor to the final product.

In a bowl, mix together the butter, salt, vanilla and sweetener. Combine well. Next, add the oats and brown rice crisps, continuing to stir with each addition. The dough should have a firm cookie dough texture. If it does not, add a little more oats or sweetener to adjust the dough. Scoop with a medium cookie scoop into balls about 1 inch in diameter. Roll in the ground nuts and set on a sheet of parchment until firm. Store in the fridge in an airtight container.

Apple (malus pumila)

An apple a day keeps the doctor away! These rose family members are well deserving of their reputation and legendary tales. Apples are chock full of nutrients including vitamins A and C, potassium, iron and fiber. The average medium apple has 5 grams of fiber, which protects against cancer and even promotes weight loss. They also offer liver support, which is linked to the tartness of the fruit. More tart apples provide more liver support. Consumption of apples on a regular basis leads to reduced cholesterol levels, improved bowel function and reduces the risk of strokes, type 2 diabetes and cancers - particularly prostate, colon and lung.

The seeds of an apple contain the same poisonous compound (amygdalin) that can be found in bitter almonds, so make sure to pull those out before handing one over to the kids. Amygdalin, when metabolized, converts to cyanide, which can cause its victims to die of asphyxiation. However, apple seeds have a hard shell, and they have to be masticated to release the amygdalin, so accidentally swallowing a seed is typically harmless. Our bodies can detoxify minor exposure to these seeds, but to err on the side of caution, it is best to remove them.

Apple butter is the yummy concentrated sauce made from apples and is a great vegan spread for morning breads. Apple cider and juices are essentially apple extracts and make a great mild laxative. (Any mom who has ever seen a two year old drink undiluted juice can attest to this one!)

Apples also make great additions to salads and flavorful sandwiches. A simple panini can be tossed together with cheddar and apples. And tart granny smith apples liven up a regular turkey sandwich. When combined with chopped peppers, onions and lime juice apples can make a yummy salsa to top chicken or the fresh cut slices can be dipped into natural peanut butter for a comfort food style snack.

Apples are typically on the "dirty dozen list" put out by the *Environmental Working Group*, which means they have some of the highest levels of pesticide residue among the foods tested, so organic apples are worth the splurge.

Medicinally, apples are great for little ones with constipation. Childhood constipation is a common concern among my clients. So many moms don't want to train their little one's bowels to rely on laxatives, yet can't seem to get them to "go" without a little assistance. Natural applesauce is a great way to boost the fiber intake and gently help things along. Here's a simple recipe that can be incorporated easily into a child's daily diet.

Natural Applesauce

Simply core and slice about 5 pounds of organic apples. Add 1/3 cup of water, place in a saucepan and cook over medium heat until soft. For smooth sauce, put through a food mill or in a processor. For chunky sauce, just stir to combine. Add 1 t cinnamon and 2-4 t honey, as desired.

Apricot (prunus armeniaca)

Apricots are loaded with vitamins A and C, fiber and potassium. These orange fruits contain phytochemicals called carotenoids, which give them their characteristic orange coloring. These antioxidants are beneficial because they help to prevent macular degeneration. When dried, apricots are a great way to get some additional iron, cobalt and copper into the diet, making them a great snack for pregnancy and / or anemia. Due to their laxative actions, dried apricots should be consumed in moderation.

Ripe apricots are quite difficult to find, partially because they do not taste good when picked unripe. Once ripened, they have a relatively short shelf life. Dried apricots are readily available and can be reconstituted for use in sauces and fillings. (To reconstitute, pour hot water over the fruit and let it sit and absorb the water.)

Fruity Apricot Vinaigrette

1 pound fresh apricots
2 T balsamic vinegar
3 T olive oil
2 t ground mustard

Chop the apricots well, then whisk in the other ingredients. The mustard helps to hold the vinaigrette together so it will not separate as quickly. If fresh apricots cannot be found, substitute 1/4 cup chopped dried apricots for the fresh and add 2 T water.

Artichoke (globe) (cynara scolymus)

There are three main types of artichokes, but most cookbooks refer to the globe variety. These thistles are native to the Mediterranean, which means that in the US, the ideal climate for them is found in California. Chock full of vitamin C, folate, magnesium, potassium, and fiber, these fat free treats also contain iron and protein.

Artichokes are also great liver tonics, as are most dark green foods. Cynarin, a phytochemical found in artichokes not only improves the liver, it also helps to lower blood cholesterol levels. In addition, artichokes aid digestion, especially the digestion of fat and they enhance the speed of blood clotting.

Our natural wellness students always become very familiar with a close cousin of artichokes, milk thistle. Milk thistle is one of my favorite herbs due to its impressive benefits on the liver, which in turn can help eliminate numerous physical ailments. Artichokes could be considered a whole food version of the herb milk thistle.

When choosing artichokes, look for heavy dark green leaves that are not turning brown or opening. To prepare the artichokes, run them under running water, cut off the stem, and remove some of the bottom leaves that are brown or separating. Steam for 45 minutes or pressure cook for about 15 minutes. Serve on a plate with a side of melted butter (feel free to add flavorful herbs to the butter). Break off a leaf, dip in the butter and put the leaf between your teeth. The filling in the outer portion of the leaf is the edible part.

Inside the choke, where the leaves are no more, is what is commonly called the heart. This can be pulled out and eaten as is, or fried in one of my favorite appetizers:

Fried Artichoke Hearts with Feta

8-10 marinated artichoke hearts
1/3 cup whole wheat bread crumbs
1 T ground seaweed (comes in a spice shaker)
dash salt and pepper
1 T Italian seasoning
1 egg
2T crumbled feta
3T Caesar dressing

Drain the hearts on a paper towel. Pour your cooking oil (coconut) into a pan and melt on medium heat. Whisk the egg. In another bowl, mix the dry ingredients. Dredge the hearts in egg then through the breadcrumbs. Drop into the oil and cook until browned (turning once), about 4 minutes.

Serve on a platter sprinkled with the feta and a bowl of Caesar dressing for dipping.

Arugula (eruca vesicaria)

Arugula, also known as rocket greens, are another Mediterranean native. They have a very slight peppery taste and can be prepared raw in salads or cooked. (Generally speaking, young greens are best in salads and older, larger ones are better cooked.) While it looks like a type of lettuce, it is actually a cruciferous vegetable, in the same family as broccoli. Aside from the calcium and vitamin C it provides, arugula also contains many valuable phytonutrients, which protect against cancer.

To add arugula to the diet, try tossing a few leaves into a salad or substituting arugula leaves for basil in your pesto. Or, try this yummy pasta

Arugula and Chevre Penne

6 ounces chevre (goat cheese), crumbled
2 cups arugula, chopped

2/3 cup sun dried tomatoes in olive oil
2 t garlic paste (or minced garlic)
dash salt and pepper

Cook 1/2 pound of penne pasta according to package directions. Drain and toss with the crumbled cheese, arugula, garlic and tomatoes. Add salt and pepper to taste and serve in 2 warm pasta dishes with crusty bread.

Asparagus (asparagus officinalis)

This vegetable is used traditionally to strengthen female reproductive organs, promote fertility, increase lactation and relieve premenstrual syndrome. When the National Cancer Institute tested a large selection of vegetables, asparagus contained the highest amount of glutathione, which is an important anti-carcinogen. Glutathione is also a mainstay in the biomedical treatments of ADHD and autism, as it plays a vital role in detoxification. Asparagus contains vitamin A, B complex vitamins, vitamin C, vitamin E, potassium and zinc.

Asparagus comes in not only the familiar green shade but also, purple and (a more expensive) white. The white is made by heaping soil above the plant, which prevents it from receiving light and making chlorophyll.

To prepare asparagus, do not cut the ends; snap them off instead. Place them in an oven proof dish, drizzle extra virgin olive oil over the top and follow with coarse sea salt. Bake at 400 degrees for 4-5 minutes. Eat them right away for a crisp, salty snack. Alternatively, cut the stalks into small segments and stir fry or sauté them. They are great added to a pasta dish in lieu of, or in addition to, meat.

The root is approved by the German Commission E for prevention of kidney stones and as a diuretic for inflammation of the urinary tract, but it is contraindicated in cases of kidney inflammation.

Avocado (Persea Americana)

Technically a fruit, avocados are commonly treated as a vegetable, mostly due to their green coloring and creamy texture. Avocados get a whopping 88% of their calories from fat, but it is a healthy monounsaturated fat, which makes them an ideal food for growing children, especially failure to thrive or other malnourished children. While adults should remember the fat content when consuming avocados, their fat should not deter a healthy adult from consuming them as part of a balanced diet. (According to the USDA, avocados contain 4.5 grams of fat per 2 tablespoons, far less than butter, which contains 23 grams, or even sour cream with 6 grams)

In addition to the healthy fats, avocados are a great source of protein, potassium, folate, vitamin E and lutein. Look for avocados that are firm, and eat them when they give lightly when pressed. My favorite way of eating avocados is in guacamole.

Homemade Guacamole

Take 1 medium avocado and cut in two. Scoop out the buttery interior, disposing of the large pit. In a small bowl, combine the pulp, 2 T fresh lemon juice, a dash of salt and pepper, 3 T of chopped tomatoes, 3 T of chopped onions, and 1/2 t ground chipotle peppers.

Mash with a fork, but do not puree. Scoop into a bowl and serve fresh with organic corn chips.

Balsamic Vinegar

While multiple imitators exist, true balsamic vinegar comes from Modena, Italy and is made from *Trebbiano* grapes. This tart yet sweet elixir is great on salads and desserts alike. When purchasing, look for true balsamic (technically, it must come from Modena) and buy the best quality you can afford. Balsamic vinegars are aged like wine, and various barrels impart differences in flavor that will vary between brands and types.

Aged balsamic is thick, almost syrupy, and is delicious with strawberries. Try mixing a little balsamic into your favorite salad dressing or dessert next time you want a healthy gourmet dinner.

Balsamic vinegar's main purpose in a whole foods diet is as a flavorful fat free contribution to our meals. Traditionally used to suppress the appetite and assist digestion, using balsamic vinegar as a topping on a first course salad takes complete advantage of all its best qualities.

As yummy as a balsamic salad may be, the recipe I'm giving you is for a luscious strawberry balsamic dessert.

Mascarpone Strawberry Balsamic Tart

Cut 6 ounces of butter into 1 3/4 cup pastry flour and 2 T sucanat. When crumbly, add 3 T ice cold water and knead until a ball is formed. Chill for an hour, then roll out onto a floured board to line a 12 inch tart pan. Poke holes in the tart with a fork and bake at 200 degrees for 20 minutes. Remove from oven and poke additional holes to vent, if needed. Stir together 2 cups fresh strawberries (diced) with 2 T aged balsamic vinegar. Set aside to mellow.

Stir together a half a pound mascarpone cheese with 1/2 t lemon essential oil. Spoon the lemon cheese mixture into the cooked tart shell and chill until dinner. Just prior to serving, spoon the strawberry mixture over the tart and serve with additional whole strawberries on the side.

Bananas (musa)

These sweet, nutritious fruits are a staple in any house with children. Bananas provide potassium, vitamin C, lutein, folate, and magnesium, containing more minerals than almost every other fruit. Their potassium content helps with hypertension and the soothing mucilage contributes to healthy digestion. While bananas are not on the "dirty dozen" list, they are often picked while still green, then sprayed with ripening agents, so organic is still the best choice. All bananas, even organic, can be found in most grocery stores year round at a great price.

Bananas are best eaten raw and fresh, but a great way to enjoy what my children often call "God's candy" is over whole grain pancakes as a fruity syrup.

1/4 pound butter (organic)
1 cup chopped nuts (optional)
3 sliced bananas
1/2 cup sucanat
1/2 cup agave nectar
1/2 cup maple syrup

Melt the butter over medium heat and add the sugars. Stir well and cook until simmering. Add the nuts and cook about 5 minutes over medium low heat. Add bananas last and stir to blend. Pour over waffles or pancakes. (Yes, this is a sugary sweet treat, great for holidays but not every day!)

Barley

With the exception of wheat, barley is one of the oldest grains. It is a common ingredient in both soup and beer, and is an acidic grain that can be made more alkaline by roasting prior to consumption. However, roasting may eliminate the laxative properties of raw barley, so that should be a consideration if medicinal benefits are expected. One half cup of cooked barley can contribute 4.5 g fiber and 12.5 mcg of folate. Barley is also great at lowering cholesterol.

Barley can be cooked into a nice side dish along other grains with wild rice or a rice blend. It can also be cooked as a risotto.

Types of barley:

- Whole barley has had its bran removed but the hull is intact. Obviously this is the highest in nutrients including protein, potassium, calcium, B vitamins and iron.
- Pearl barley has lost its bran, fiber, B vitamins and many of its minerals. While it is one of the most readily available forms of barley, it is much less nutritious.
- Barley flour can be used in breads for a portion of the flour. It is naturally low in gluten, making it a healthy addition, but also making it more difficult for baking lighter, fluffier breads.
- Barley grass is the chlorophyll laden grass than is commonly juiced for its high concentration of nutrients.

Barley Risotto makes a great side dish or light meal full of nutrients. This recipe is a family favorite and a great introduction of the grain to new palates.

1 pound whole barley
4 cups chicken broth (organic or homemade to avoid MSG)
2 cups water
2 T olive oil
1/4 cup chopped carrots
1/4 cup green peas
1/4 cup diced onions
1/4 cup zucchini, cut into cubes
1/2 t garlic puree

Heat the olive oil over medium heat. Add the barley and toast gently. Add 1/2 t garlic puree, stir well, and add the onions and 1 cup of the broth. Simmer until the broth is absorbed. Continue adding the liquids 1 cup at a time, only adding more as the previous addition is almost absorbed. When all the liquid is almost absorbed (about 15 minutes), add 1 T butter and 2-3 T grated cheese (ideally a hard Italian cheese.) Serve immediately.

Beans

Anyone who has memorized popular grade school songs can tell you that beans contribute a very high amount of fiber to the diet. This vegetarian protein source is also high in phytochemicals like diosgenin, which inhibits cancer. Beans also reduce cholesterol and are typically high in calcium, potassium, iron, zinc, B vitamins and magnesium. Beans also contain isoflavones, which prevent cancer and heart disease.

Beans and grains go together well to form a complete protein. While food combining is not a necessity for healthy lifestyles, it does simplify things for those who are concentrating on obtaining more varied sources of protein to be aware what types of amino acids are in common foods.. To lower the "magical-ness" of beans, soak them well prior to cooking. Depending on the bean, 6-12 hours are typically sufficient. This activates enzymes that begin to digest the carbohydrates into starches that are much easier for our bodies to digest. Preprocessed beans and canned beans do not have the important B vitamins that are found in dried beans.

Note: Some food guides list beans as a food to avoid when taking medications that are MAO inhibitors.

Hummus is a great way to get a little extra protein into kids and serving them with pitas gives them a great protein variety. Try dipping carrots and other veggies as well.

2 cups dried chickpeas
1 T pureed garlic
1 t salt
2/3 cup tahini
1/4 cup fresh lemon juice
4-5 T olive oil
1/2 cup water or chicken broth

Soak and cook the beans, Place into a food processor with the garlic, salt, tahini, lemon oil and water or broth. OPTIONAL: Add 1/4 cup roasted red peppers. Process until smooth. Add fresh or dried parsley and serve with pita chips.

Beef

Beef is a great source of B vitamins, iron, phosphorus, zinc and beneficial fatty acids known as CLAs, which inhibit cancer. Beef can also be a source of saturated fat and cholesterol. The best way to consume beef is from free range, grass fed cattle that have not been raised with hormones or antibiotics, fully cooked, and combined with vitamin C, which aids in the absorption of iron.

While the topic of eating meat can be somewhat controversial in the holistic health realm, I have yet to find a good reason to avoid healthy meats. As mentioned in the protein section earlier, meats are not the ideal center of every meal, but 2-4 times a week enables one to benefit from the nutrients to be found, while still preventing the ill effects of over-consumption.

It is very important to focus on grass fed beef. Grass fed beef is ideal because it contains higher amounts of omega 3s, more CLAs (conjugated dienole linoleic acid) and vitamin E. If making the switch, you will need to learn how to cook grass fed beef, as it requires different methods. You also may need to adjust to the taste, although many people do not notice a difference.

Steak kabobs combine the iron and B vitamins with vitamin C, making them a great meal for anemia - and a great snack for pregnant mamas!

1 sirloin steak, chopped into large cubes
1 each red and green peppers, sliced
1 onion, chopped into large chunks
pineapple cubes (optional)
salt and pepper to taste
fresh rosemary spring

Slide the cubes onto a skewer, alternating between steak and veggies. Add the pineapple into the mix, if using. Top with a rosemary sprig and grill over medium-high heat until desired level of doneness is achieved. Serve over a bed of wild and brown rice.

Beer

Beer is a fermented beverage made by yeasts that have converted the sugars found in malted barley and other grains to alcohol (ethyl alcohol). The USDA defines one beer as 12 ounces. Traditionally considered to be "empty calories," beer actually retains many of the nutrients formally found in the ingredients that were brewed. Additionally, locally brewed beers (and homebrewed beers) are often healthier and have a more diverse ingredient list than mass market beers.

Beer is rich in folate, niacin, magnesium, phosphorus and vitamin B6. Studies from the American Cancer Society show that men who take one drink a day have a lower risk of heart attack and stroke (21% and 22% lower, respectively) then men who did not drink at all. Alcohol also decreases the body's production of, and storage of, LDL. People who drink moderate amounts of alcohol tend to have lower levels of LDL and higher levels of HDL. USDA guidelines of moderate consumption are 2 drinks a day for men and 1 a day for women.

However, higher amounts increase the risk of many cancers, according to the American Cancer Society. Pregnant women who drink 2 or more drinks a day increase the risk of fetal alcohol syndrome, though there is no evidence of a consistent pattern of birth defects in women who consume less than 1 alcoholic drink a day.

Alcoholic drinks can also create a dependence known as alcoholism, rounder bellies (beer bellies), and a burden on the liver. For this reason, milk thistle or dandelion supplementation is often recommended for those who consume beer regularly. There is no included recipe for beer; it is typically consumed as-is.

Beets

These bright colored veggies are loaded with vitamin C and potassium. One serving of beets contains 33% of the RDA for folate and 27% of the RDA for manganese. Beets are also high in iron, fiber and magnesium.

Beets are not only good for treating anemia; they also prevent and inhibit cancer. They contain betacyanin, a powerful cancer fighting pigment. Beets increase the body's production of glutathione and protect the liver from attacks by free radicals. Since the liver is our detox organ, beets contribute to detoxification of the body. Because of this, many natural cancer therapies include fresh beet juice in their treatments.

Introducing beets to the diet may result in pink tinged urine or stool. This is common and will pass. Too many beets in the diet can also cause health problems in persons with kidney or gallbladder problems due to the high oxalate content.

Studies show that the anti cancer properties in beets are destroyed by heat, so the best way to eat them is lightly cooked or juiced. Beets can also change colors due to the pH of the other ingredients in a dish. For optimal cancer fighting properties, try beets raw, as in this salad.

Red and Green Salad

2 T Dijon mustard
2 T apple cider vinegar
2 T olive oil
salt and pepper to taste
2-3 granny smith apples
1/4 cup dried cranberries
1/4 cup slivered almonds
1 cup raw beets, peeled and grated
2 ounces crumbled feta
2 cups baby greens

In a small bowl, whisk together the first 5 ingredients to make a vinaigrette. Set aside. Toss together the greens with the cranberries, apples, almonds, beets and feta. Serve with the vinaigrette.

Blackberries (rubus ulmfolius)

Nothing reminds me of summer more than big juicy berries. These antioxidant rich fruits are mild diuretics and astringent in action. In addition, blackberries offer vitamins A, C, E and K, folate, copper, calcium and manganese.

The dark pigments in berries provide the powerful antioxidants in the fruits, which are good for fighting free radicals in the body. Berries should be kept in the fridge and eaten quickly since they do not last long.

Blackberries are best eaten raw, as cooking destroys much of the vitamin C and lets the water soluble B vitamins leak out. Their leaves however can be brewed into a tea, which is useful for diarrhea and mild inflammation of the throat.

To treat diarrhea, try this yummy, hydrating tea: Combine 2 t blackberry leaves with a cup of boiling water. Steep 5 minutes then strain. Add 2 T mashed and strained fresh blackberries. Enjoy

Black Eyed Peas

Growing up in Alabama, black eyed peas were a staple at my grandmother's table. To this day, I am served a huge portion of creamed corn (the yummy natural kind) and black eyed peas (also known as field peas) every time I head down for a visit. These legumes are a great source of protein and fiber.

While my grandmother's famous black eyed peas used ham hocks for a traditional flavor, I like to spice things up a bit with a portable black eyed pea fritter.

Black Eyed Pea Fritters

2 cups cooked black eyed peas
2 eggs, beaten
1/2 cup flour, any type
1 small onion, chopped into small pieces
1 minced clove garlic
1/2 t baking powder (aluminum free)
1 t salt
pepper, to taste

Combine all ingredients in a large bowl. Lightly mash the peas just enough to keep the mixture together, without turning into mush. Shape into small discs, about 2 inches in diameter. Fry in hot oil, about 350 degrees, turning once, until golden brown. This should take about 1-2 minutes per side.

Blueberries

Blueberries have a great reputation as a health food due to their high antioxidant content. Nutritionally, blueberries are a great source of vitamins C and A as well as manganese. Medicinally, blueberries support healthy eye function and help fight urinary tract infections, as do their cousins, cranberries. Blueberries also help reduce the risk of heart disease, cancer, dementia, and other aging related troubles. These properties are often attributed to their high antioxidant content. Allergic reactions are fairly common however, as berries are among the twelve most common allergens.

Blueberries can be purchased fresh in the produce section. They do not last long, but they freeze well. This makes them great for smoothies and tossing into breakfast batters (waffle and pancake work well). For an antioxidant boost and to support healthy eye function, try this breakfast smoothie.

Antioxidant Berry Smoothie

2 cups frozen berries (blueberries, blackberries, raspberries)
1 banana
1/2 cup orange juice

Blend 2-3 minutes until smooth. Optional: Add 2-3 T flax seed oil. Serve immediately.

Broccoli

Loaded with calcium, folate, vitamin C, selenium, vitamin A, vitamin E, and fiber, broccoli is a highly nutritious kid friendly vegetable. A fresh cooked broccoli spear contains as much as 5 grams of fiber and over half of the RDA for folate and vitamins A and C.

The best way to eat broccoli is raw, as this eliminates the chance of nutrient loss during the cooking process. Broccoli sprouts are a great way to take advantage of the potent cancer fighting compounds and obtain the most available nutrients.

For a fiber boost, try this quick and easy recipe: Take about 2 cups broccoli heads, wash and chop in half, then place in a baking dish. Drizzle olive oil over the top, add a dash salt and pepper and then sprinkle with hard Italian cheese (about 1/2 cup) Bake in a 400 degree oven 10-15 minutes, enough to melt the cheese but not make the broccoli soggy. Serve immediately.

Brussels Sprouts

Another green vegetable, Brussels sprouts, provides many of the same nutrients broccoli does. You can expect to gain vitamins A and C, folate, potassium, iron and fiber from a plate of this veggie. Brussels sprouts also contain an anti-nutrient; this mineral splits the vitamin B1 (thiamin) molecule so it is no longer useful. Cooking the sprouts can deactivate this anti-nutrient. The best way to eat Brussels sprouts is by lightly steaming them, which will destroy the anti-nutrient, retaining many of the vitamins.

The naturally-occurring, anti-cancer compounds in Brussels sprouts make them a great side dish to any meal. Slightly sweet, they combine well with the tangy Dijon mustard, as in this recipe:

Dijon Brussels Sprouts: Boil 1 pound Brussels sprouts in a pot of water until tender, about 5-10 minutes. Drain. Add to a pan with 1-2T olive oil and sauté 4-5 minutes. Add 3 T Dijon mustard and a dash of sea salt, pepper and dried parsley. Stir until well combined. Scoop into a shallow dish.

Bulgur

Bulgur is actually a dish, not a food. Basically, it is composed of steamed, dried and cracked whole wheat. To make bulgur, soak a cup of whole wheat overnight, then drain. Place berries and 2 cups of water in a covered pan, and simmer for about 45 minutes. Drain again, place on a baking sheet and place in a warm oven (about 200 degrees) for an hour. Once it's dry, blend it in the blender and store in the pantry.

Basil Pecan Bulgur: For a great high protein dish, take 1 cup of bulgur; toss with 1 T chopped fresh basil, 1 T rosemary, and a dash of salt. Place them into a shallow baking dish with 2 cups of water. Bake, covered at 250 degrees for 15 to 20 minutes. Add 1/4 to 1/3 cup whole pecans, fluff with a fork and serve immediately.

Butter

Butter is great for cooking foods at high heat. Organic butter made from free range, grass fed, antibiotic and hormone free cows or goats is the healthiest type of butter to consume. Since butter is the concentrated fat from dairy, and mammals tend to store toxins in fat, it is important to make sure to obtain a quality product. Butter comes in two forms, salted and unsalted. Most culinary professionals agree unsalted is best for baking and candy making. Salted is best used as a table butter (i.e.: buttering bread). In addition to pure butter, ghee can be derived from butter. Ghee is essentially clarified butter. It is a staple in Eastern cooking, and effective at both easing digestion and preventing cancer. You can purchase ghee at a health food store or make your own.

Homemade Ghee

Take a pound of butter, put it into a medium pan and bring to a boil. Reduce heat to medium. Foam will form, then disappear. When the second foam appears, scrape it off, then gently pour the top of the solids off into your container. Be sure to leave the milks solids in the pan. Ghee does not need to be refrigerated and will keep up to a month.

Cabbage

Not only does it attract baby bunny rabbits, cabbage is packed with vitamins C and K, fiber, omega 3s, calcium, folate and manganese. Like broccoli and Brussels sprouts, cabbage is high in cancer fighting compounds. Cabbage is best eaten raw, as in its most popular dish, slaw. Another healthy way of consuming cabbage is to make sauerkraut. This fermented dish is immersed in a salt solution that is strong enough to kill off harmful bacteria, but still allows the beneficial strands to survive, which then break down the proteins in the cabbage. Sauerkraut is much higher in sodium and lower in vitamins than raw cabbage, so keep that in mind as well.

In addition to the supply of vitamins and nutrients, cabbage is a good cleanser for the body and supports healthy digestion and female health. My absolute favorite way to enjoy cabbage is in cabbage rolls.

Cabbage Rolls

Simply take any leftover meat (chicken is ideal) and add chopped veggies with loads of flavor such as peppers. Stir together over medium heat with a little water and seasonings (onion, garlic) spoon into a cool crisp cabbage shell, fold over and enjoy.

Capers (capparis spinosa)

Capers are harvested from a bush in the Mediterranean and placed in brine for storage. As well as imparting great flavor to Mediterranean dishes, capers are great for the digestive tract, especially in the case of diarrhea.

Capers are high in sodium and do not contribute much of any particular nutrient, but are good at what they do, which is flavoring food. Try adding them to your favorite Mediterranean dish, or try this digestion promoting recipe:

Chicken with artichokes and capers

8 thin chicken breasts
1/3 cup fresh whole wheat flour, mixed with salt, pepper and garlic powder
Juice of 2 whole lemons
1/2 cup white wine
1/2 cup chicken broth (or sub 1 whole cup and omit the wine, if preferred)
1/4 cup capers
8-10 artichoke hearts

Dredge the chicken in the flour mixture, then sauté in butter over medium heat until browned. (Since they are so thin, they should cook quickly.) Once cooked (about 5 minutes) remove and keep warm. Add the wine (if using) broth and juice to the pan and stir well. Cook about 5 minutes until it has thickened. Add the capers to the sauce and cook an additional minute or two. Remove from heat, add the artichokes and serve the chicken over a bed of wild and brown rice topped with the artichoke and caper sauce.

Carob

Carob is a legume native to the Mediterranean. Rich in calcium (it contains more than milk), potassium, vitamins A and B, carob is also a great source of protein and is free of caffeine.

Carob is most known, however, as a substitute for chocolate. Most health food stores have a wide variety of carob options from powder to chips and drinks. This is one of the unfortunate cases of "the health food store carries it so it must be better" mindset. Yes, carob is caffeine free, but caffeine is not the villain it has been made out to be. Most of the health problems with chocolate stem from the sugar and dairy that is added during processing

That being said, carob is an extremely nutritional food and makes a great addition to the diet, especially for those allergic to chocolate or on an anti-fungal diet. Chocolate also is a common allergen and carob makes a great option for those individuals. For a little variety in the diet, try these carob nut snacks, which are high in protein, making them great for growing children.

2 cups carob chips
2/3 cup nut butter (peanut or almond)
1 T vanilla extract (not artificial vanilla)
1 cup assorted nuts (try varying or complimenting the butter)
1 1/2 cup oats

Over the stove, melt the chips with the nut butter and vanilla. Once thinned, stir in the nuts and oats. When combined, scoop into clusters on a sheet of parchment paper and let harden. (Note: These will resemble "no bake" style cookies, but with less sugar and tons of great protein and nutrients.)

Carrot

Carrots are one of our most common and valuable vegetables. Not only do they transport easily, they have a great shelf life and are packed with nutrients. The average carrot provides lycopene, vitamin A and B complex, carotenoids, phosphorus and calcium. Carrots help to cleanse the body and their fresh juice is a staple in many natural cancer remedies.

They earn their cleansing reputation due to their supportive effect on the liver and kidneys, combined with their diuretic effect, which helps to eliminate excess fluid. Their fiber helps to prevent constipation, which also contributes to the cleansing effect. Carrots contain a phenol, coumarin, which thins the blood, preventing clots. With all the cleansing action and healthy fiber, carrots are perfect for both preventing and fighting cancer.

The best way to eat a carrot is raw. Carrots can be added to salads, eaten as snacks and as a side dish to a meal. Since they are firm and do not damage easily, they are perfect for travel and in kid's lunch boxes.

Carrots are rich in sugar, so their juice contains less fiber and more sugar than eating them whole. To observe a strict whole foods diet, the whole carrot would be eaten, not just the juice, however fresh it may be. Still, carrot juice is a great source of nutrients, especially in a body that is in a less than optimal state of health.

While the best way to consume carrots is fresh and raw, many picky eaters don't particularly care! This is when a little clever kitchen creativity comes in handy. For the picky eater, try this yummy cupcake recipe, which sneaks in a few good nutrients.

Carrot Cupcakes

1 pound grated carrots
2 cups whole wheat flour
1 t each: cinnamon, salt, baking soda and powder
4 large eggs
1 cup sucanat
1 cup agave nectar
1/4 cup (1/2 stick) butter, softened
1 t real vanilla
1/3 cup cream cheese, softened
1 t real vanilla
1/2 cup honey

Mix dry ingredients together and set aside. In another bowl, beat the eggs, then add the sucanat, butter, carrots, and vanilla. Slowly add the dry ingredients. Once combined (do not over mix), scoop into prepared muffin cups (fill 2/3 full). Bake at 325 for 18-20 minutes. Let cool.

Combine the cream cheese with the honey and vanilla. Be sure the mixture is fully combined. Spread over cooled cupcakes and serve immediately or store in the fridge.

Cashew

This Brazil native naturally comes encased in a shell, which contains oil with properties similar to those of poison ivy. For this reason, these nuts are pre-shelled, then roasted twice to remove all traces of the oil before they are sold.

These nuts are lower in fat than most other nuts, and rich in protein, potassium, phosphorus and magnesium. You will find these nuts sold as "raw" in the grocery store, which simply means they have not been roasted further. They are also common in a wide amount of Eastern dishes. I enjoy cashews in yummy, kid friendly pesto dip.

Cashew Pesto Dip

1 T pureed garlic
1 cup basil leaves
1 T dried parsley
1/4 cup extra virgin olive oil
1 cup roasted cashews

Place all ingredients into a food processor or blender. Puree. Scoop into a dipping bowl, top with a grated hard cheese and serve with toasted slices of crusty bread.

Cauliflower

Cauliflower is packed with vitamins C and B complex, as well as fiber, potassium, and calcium. These creamy colored veggies also offer protection against cancer, as they contain naturally occurring antioxidants.

In addition to serving raw with a dip, as is cauliflower's usual fare, the nutritious benefits can also be obtained in this savory gratin.

Cauliflower Gratin

Take 1-2 heads of cauliflower, wash, and chop them into chunks. Place in a casserole dish. Stir together 1/2 t pureed garlic with 2-3 T of extra virgin olive oil and drizzle the mixture on top. Add a dash of salt and white pepper. Bake at 375 degrees for 15-20 minutes until the florets are nice and lightly browned. Remove and cover with a grated hard cheese, then serve immediately.

Celery

Celery is another extremely common vegetable. Who doesn't have fond memories of "ants on a log" made with raisins, peanut butter and celery? In addition to functioning as a "log," celery adds the perfect extra crunch on a salad or in soups.

Celery provides fiber, folate, potassium and phosphorus to the diet and is low in fat and calories. The fiber and vitamins help to lower the risk of cancer and prevent constipation.

Since celery has more crunch than flavor, I love to add it to a raw food salad. Try this nutrient rich and flavorful recipe for lunch or a light evening meal.

Green Salad with Celery and Maple Glazed Pecans

Toss together the following:
3 cups organic baby greens
2 granny smith apples, cored and diced
1/4 cup dried cranberries
5-7 stalks of celery, diced
5-6 cherry tomatoes

Place in a large serving bowl. Place 1/4 cup pecans and 2 T maple syrup in a saucepan. Cook over medium heat about 5 minutes until the syrup forms a crisp crust on the pecans. Remove from heat and toss onto the salad with 3-4 T of bleu cheese. Douse with balsamic vinaigrette.

Chard

Chard is a close relative to beets. It comes in both red and white and the leaves are either wavy or flat. Huge clumps of bright red chard are always the first thing I see in my weekly CSA box in the spring months.

Like most leafy greens, chard supports the liver, prevents constipation, boosts the blood and is a great source of chlorophyll, vitamins K, A, and

C, magnesium, manganese, potassium and iron. One cup of chard (175g) supplies over 700% of the RDA of vitamin K! The anthocyanins in chard (which are phytonutrients) help to prevent cancers of the digestive tract, especially colon cancer. The beta carotene helps support healthy eyes, and the magnesium helps to balance calcium in the body.

Chard is actually not native to Switzerland, but it was discovered by a Swiss botanist, and thus named for his homeland. In keeping with the trend of other nutrient dense foods, chard is actually a native to the Mediterranean region.

Chard is best cooked, either steamed or sautéed, as in this recipe:

Take 2 large bunches of chard, wash and cut into 1 inch strips. Set aside. In a saucepan, place 2-3 T olive oil, 1 T pureed garlic, and a dash of red pepper flakes (optional) Once hot, add the chard and quickly combine. Cook, stirring occasionally, for 6-8 minutes then serve immediately.

Cheese

Cheese is a fairly general term for any curdled milk. Cheese can be made from cow, goat, sheep or other mammals' milk. When cheese is made, the milk protein (casein) is broken in half. One half becomes a solid mass (the curds) and the other is the cheese making by-product also known as whey. Cheese is considered to be a healthier way of consuming dairy, because it is fermented or partially digested prior to consumption. This makes the job much easier on our digestive systems.

Cheeses come in a wide range of types and flavors. All cheese should be a creamy white color naturally. The flavors depend upon the type of milk used, the length of time fermented and aged, and the method of cheese making. Cheese making, like wine making is a very defined art, and artisan cheeses are generally well worth their price.

While those with a true milk allergy must avoid dairy cheese, many who are intolerant to dairy can tolerate cheese or yogurt, as the proteins have been altered and the actual finished substance is quite different. For others who are allergic or intolerant to cow milk products, goat's milk cheese is a viable alternative. Goat's milk can be made into many of the same cheeses that cow's milk is made into.

Obviously, the nutrient content of cheese will vary drastically according to which method and type of milk is used. However, generalities can still be made. Cheese is generally rich in calcium, phosphorus, riboflavin, protein, zinc, and even fat.

Due to the fact that cheese is an animal product and generally high in fat, it is best and most often used as a condiment. Sprinkled over nutritious veggies or pasta, the tangy and savory taste can shine, while the fat is kept to a minimum. Every so often, however, a good cheese deserves a starring role in a recipe, especially if it is my personal favorite: a fresh, high quality tangy goat cheese - absolutely delicious!

To see what I mean, try this **bruschetta**:

Take a 4 ounce log of good quality chevre. Slice it into 8 rounds. In a shallow dish, pour 1.5 cups of your favorite tomato pasta sauce. Top with rounds of cheese. Place into a 400 degree oven. Meanwhile, slice a baguette into 1 inch slices. Rub with garlic and lightly toast. Remove the dish from the oven. Stir to combine (it will turn orange). Spoon over the toast slices. Serve as an appetizer or snack.

Cherries

Cherries are the sweet relatives of plums, known for their tolerance to cold and sweet or tart flavors. These bright red stone fruits are a lush source of iron, vitamin A, phosphorus, calcium and potassium.

Cherries, like many foods, are best eaten raw. Look for them in their prime season, which is midsummer. They don't last long, and they do not travel well, but they can be found frozen in health foods stores year round. The frozen fruits can be baked in to pies and other treats, adding a tangy kick and boost of iron and vitamins.

To best take advantage of frozen cherries, try them in this yummy cherry sorbet:

Take 3 cups of frozen cherries and mix in a medium saucepan with 1/2 cup of water and 1/3 cup of sucanat. Stir well while you bring it to a boil. Simmer about 5 minutes, then remove and let cool. Puree in a food processor. (If desired, at this point, strain to remove the skin) Mix with 3 T fresh lime juice and pour into an ice cream maker, following the maker's directions.

Chick Peas

Chickpeas (garbanzo beans) have been enjoyed since the days of ancient Greece and Rome. These Mediterranean natives are the most widely consumed legumes in the world, for good reason. Not only are they loaded with fiber and protein, they provide manganese, folate, copper, phosphorus and iron. One cup of chickpeas offers 70% of the RDA for folate and 85% of the RDA for manganese. The same size serving would also provide 12.5 grams of fiber and 14.5 grams of protein.

The best way to consume these legumes is to first soak them about 12 hours, then strain off the liquid. After adding fresh water, cook 1.5 hours then add salt and pepper to taste. The most popular way of eating chickpeas is in the dish hummus.

Chili Peppers

Chili pepper is the name given to an entire group of peppers. As one of the most common condiments, they earn their popularity from their heat. These spicy peppers increase blood circulation, increase the body temperature and can even cause perspiration, conversely cooling the body back down.

Contraindicated for those with inflamed colons, peppers stimulate the digestive system and have valuable antioxidant properties. Due to the irritating factor from the capsicum contained in peppers, they should be handled with gloves and never allowed in the eyes.

Peppers are traditionally used in savory entrees for lunch and dinner, but they can be used for breakfast with potatoes as in this recipe:

2.5 pounds of red potatoes, washed and sliced
3 T oil
1 onion, chopped
1 cup assorted peppers (as hot or cool as you like them) chopped
dash salt and pepper

Toss all ingredients together. Bake at 350 degrees for 15 minutes or until soft. Transfer to a greased pan over medium high heat. Finish cooking on the stove, searing the edges to a golden brown crisp (about 3 minutes).

Chocolate

This enticing substance has had its ups and downs throughout history. The ancient bean was exalted in the Mayan culture as a fertility booster and exotic fare for the wealthy and privileged. In 1492, on his return from America, Columbus brought back cocoa beans, but they were largely ignored by the King and Queen. Fortunately, Fernando Cortez discovered that by adding sugar this unfamiliar drink could become a delicacy. In 1830, the drink became a real treat, as the first solid chocolate was created.

Unfortunately, as of late, chocolate has become so adulterated with additives that it earned a bad reputation as a high fat and high calorie food. To our rescue comes modern science by letting us know just how great this food really is. Loaded with valuable nutrients, this once forbidden food has again earned its place as a healthy but luxurious delight.

Of course, the only healthy chocolate is natural dark chocolate, not the grocery store variety that is mostly milk, sugar and artificial vanilla. Real, unadulterated chocolate is the truly good stuff.

This real chocolate contains antioxidants in numbers that make red wine and green tea pale in comparison. Antioxidants are substances that protect our bodies from potential damage done by free radicals. By protecting us from free radicals, antioxidants can prevent or slow cancer in our bodies. Antioxidant capacity is measured by ORAC units (Oxygen Radical Absorption Capacity). Dark chocolate contains over 13,000 ORAC units.

The benefits don't end there. It turns out that chocolate is actually good for the heart as well. The same flavonols help to prevent fat like substances in the blood stream from clogging the arteries. According to a recent study, these flavonols prevent clotting as well as a dose of aspirin. They keep the blood flowing well by preventing the platelets from sticking together, which in turn prevents arteries from clogging.

Furthermore, the boost you feel after eating a piece of chocolate is not a product of your imagination! Real chocolate contains tryptophan, the famous amino acid we remember from the Thanksgiving turkey. This relieves stress, as does the body's own endorphins, which are released through chocolate consumption. It is also a natural analgesic and anti-inflammatory.

To quote a recently published study, "The benefits of chocolate can be enjoyed without guilt as part of a healthful balanced diet." Yep, you read it correctly: without guilt. In all fairness, I should note that the benefits are not in chocolate syrup or other modified sources. The antioxidant properties are in cocoa and dark chocolate and, to a lesser extent, in milk chocolate. The other nutritional benefits are found primarily in dark chocolate. I suggest purchasing only the best natural and organic chocolate available for maximum health benefits, and obviously, moderation is the key. Cocoa butter is still a high fat substance and should not be consumed without regard to the saturated fat involved. The suggested amount is 2 ounces a day with a minimum of 70% cocoa content.

Here's a great way to get started with this new guilt free indulgence:

Crunchy Chocolate Truffles

1 cup almond, hazelnut or other natural nut butter
3/4 cup of dark chocolate bits
1 cup oats, puffed millet, or brown rice crisps (available at a health food store)
1/2 cup chopped nuts (preferably the same kind as the butter)
optional: 1/2 cup of grated chocolate

Place the nut butter and nuts in a saucepan over medium heat until softened (or zap in the microwave for about 30 to 45 seconds). Add the chocolate bits and stir until softened. Quickly, stir in the grains (using one or a combo the three to make up 2/3 cup) Stir until combined. Roll into 1 inch balls and set on waxed paper until firm. Roll in the grated chocolate for a gourmet touch. Store in the fridge for up to a week. Serve cooled or at room temperature.

Citrus Fruits

Citrus fruits, in general, are alkalizing, tangy and full of nutrients, especially vitamin C. Oranges, lemons and limes are the most common fruits, but tangerines, passion fruit and even kumquats fall under this grouping.

Oranges are rich in vitamins, with one medium orange offering close to 70% of the RDA for vitamin C. They also offer fiber, folate, vitamin B1, potassium, vitamin A, and even calcium. Over 60 flavonoids have been found in oranges, providing powerful antioxidant and anti-inflammatory protection.

Orange juice, the most common breakfast juice, is a great way to obtain many of the benefits of oranges, but it is important to keep in mind that this forfeits most of the fiber, and the juice itself is a sugary, somewhat processed food. (One orange offers over 3 grams of fiber or 13% of the RDA.) The best juice to drink would be fresh and consuming the whole fruit is even better.

Many experts will list citrus fruits as a food that does not *have* to be purchased organic. While it is true that peeling the fruit can eliminate many of the residues, we need to be especially aware of citrus zests, peels, and oils. These should be organic, as they come from the peel, which contains this potent concentration of toxic residues. This is especially important in light of some recent research showing that the peels of citrus fruits are a concentrated source of polymethoxylated flavones, which may have the power to lower cholesterol better than some prescription drugs. To obtain these flavones, citrus zest and peel can be added to treats that contain citrus.

Lemons and limes are also nutrient powerhouses, offering nearly half the RDA of vitamin C and plenty of carotenoids and flavonoids. As oranges, lemons and limes are best consumed raw; I like to keep sliced lemons in the fridge to add to my water both for flavor and for its alkalizing abilities.

For a vitamin C boost, or just a yummy dessert, try this citrus blend: Take 4 oranges and chop them into cubes. Place in a serving dish with 2 cups of strawberries, hulled and halved. In another bowl, whisk together the fresh juice of 1 lemon and lime, the zest of the lemon and limes, and 3 T raw honey. Pour the sauce over the fruit and serve chilled.

Coconut (Oil)

This tropical food has multiple uses and travels well. The forms of coconut readily available to us are the oil and the dried pulp, and the two offer different health benefits.

Coconut oil is a saturated fat from the coconut itself. This oil is solid at most room temperatures, making it ideal for transporting. (Coconut oil typically melts at 76 degrees) In the low fat days, coconut oil dropped dramatically in popularity despite the oil's convenience, simply because it was saturated. It was usually replaced by "healthier" hydrogenated oils.

Recent studies, however, show us that the proverbial baby was tossed out with the bath water. Coconut oil only contains 9% of the long chain fatty acids (palmatic acid), which are the type implicated in heart disease. Two thirds of the saturated fats in coconut oil are medium chain fatty acids in the form of caprylic, capric and lauric acids. Lauric acid has actually gained a reputation as a heart protective acid. Similar acids have long been used to aid in digestion and absorption. Coconut oil can be assumed to provide many of the same benefits, since it contains similar types of acids.

If you spend much time online, you can also find information promoting coconut oil as antiviral, antibacterial, a weight loss aid, and overall health miracle. While coconut oil does contain many compounds with antiviral and antibacterial benefits, some of the outlandish claims are speculation and cannot be substantiated.

To give coconut oil a try, use it in place of solid oils in recipes, or try popping popcorn in coconut oil over the stove. Obviously virgin coconut oil is the best, but refined can be used when the mild coconut oil taste is not needed.

Coffee

This morning beverage is another example of a regular food with a bad reputation. While most people will admit to drinking coffee, most also believe it is a bad habit in need of breaking. Coffee is a diuretic drink, as most can attest to. It offers a boost of caffeine, which stimulates the nervous system, stresses the adrenal glands and elevates blood pressure. It can also decrease the absorption of minerals, depleting the body of B complex and calcium.

Yet, coffee is the greatest source of antioxidants found in the average diet. To give you an idea of how many antioxidants can be found, the average adult consumes 1299 mg of antioxidants daily from coffee. The closest competitor is tea with 294 mg. In addition, the National Cancer Institute found that those that consumed coffee daily had half the risk of liver cancer compared to those that never drank it. The Harvard School of Public health found that men who drank more than six 8 ounce cups daily cut their chance of diabetes by half and women by 30%. (Of course, six cups of coffee would provide more risks than benefits, so it is not recommended!)

Corn

Corn, maize, whatever you prefer, this ancient food packs a punch. While rich in B1, folate, fiber, vitamin C, phosphorus and manganese, corn has a glycemic index of 78, making it a sugary sweet treat as well. When eating corn, the white varieties of corn are a tad sweeter, making the yellow version, with lots of healthy carotenoids, the healthier pick. Yellow corn also boasts vitamin A and beta carotene, which is absent in white corn.

This sweet food, however, is not without its caveats. Corn is a naturally rich source of oxalates and is a common allergen.

Other methods of consuming corn include corn meal (which is dried ground corn), corn grits or polenta (which are essentially the same food, only cooked differently), and corn chips or tortillas (which are made from corn mesa). These methods of preparing corn still hold many, but not all of the nutrients found in fresh corn.

The nutrient offerings of corn offer many benefits, such as increased energy production, lung health, and powerful antioxidant activity. The best way to eat corn is not boiled, as so commonly done. Boiling any vegetable allows nutrients to leach out into the water, which is often discarded. For best nutrient retention, try grilling, broiling or steaming vegetables, as this assures most of the nutrients remain with the food. For another way to prepare corn, try my Grandmother's famous creamed corn, an original whole food!

Naturally Creamed Corn

Simply take 4-6 ears of corn (raw) and literally shave the kernels off into a pan. As they come off, you will notice a naturally occurring creamy substance. Place the pan over heat and cook about 10 minutes. Add butter and salt to taste, stirring regularly. My grandmother used to buy large amounts of corn from local farmers every summer and make huge batches of creamed corn. She would then measure them out by the cup and freeze it in meal-sized portions. Every time we came to visit, we knew we would eat "vegetables" for dinner, which featured her famous creamed corn and black-eyed peas. She was an original locally grown whole foods enthusiast!

Couscous

Couscous is the light, fluffy miniature pasta popular in Middle Eastern dishes. It is generally made from durum wheat, but in some places millet couscous can be found. The health benefits will be consistent with the grain from which it is made.

When purchasing couscous, I do not recommend the boxed and flavored kind. These typically contain MSG or a version of it. Plain couscous can be purchased for much less, and you can alter it to match your fare. Try this recipe for **couscous with sun dried tomatoes and basil**.

1 T olive oil
1/2 cup sliced scallions
1 t pureed garlic
2 cups chicken broth and 1 cup water
1/2 t dried basil
1 1/2 cups couscous
1/4 cup marinated chopped sun dried tomatoes
dash salt and pepper

Place all ingredients in a medium saucepan over medium heat. Bring to a boil. Remove from heat, cover and let sit 12 minutes. Stir to combine and serve hot.

Cranberry

This Thanksgiving classic, which was widely enjoyed by the Native Americans, is a nutrient rich gem. Cranberry's medical history includes being used in poultices for wounds (cranberries are rich in astringent tannins) and as a daily vitamin source. These tart red berries are rich in vitamin C, fiber and manganese, but their real power is in the mega amounts of antioxidants naturally occurring in the fruit.

You are probably familiar with cranberries from their other medicinal use, preventing and treating urinary tract infections. The berries contain a substance called hippuric acid, which is antibacterial. It also contains substances that inhibit *E coli,* which is the main cause of urinary tract infections. Additionally, the berries inhibit the ability of the bacteria to stick to the urinary tract, which reduces the chance of infection.

The berries also contain quinic acid, which helps to prevent kidney stones from forming. The antioxidants benefit the heart health and the *E coli* prevention also helps to inhibit other related *E coli* problems such as food poisoning.

The best way to eat cranberries, as most foods, is fresh. While fresh berries last quite awhile, many of us can only get our hands on frozen or dried fruits. The berries still retain many of their nutrients when frozen or dried. Dried cranberries are an ideal source of nutrients, since the main contribution is in the form of antioxidants, not vitamin C, which is lost in the drying process, and dried cranberries are often consumed raw, whereas frozen berries are often cooked, which destroys many nutrients.

Another great way to enjoy raw berries is in a berry salsa, like this one:

Cranberry Salsa

1 orange, chopped finely
4 cups fresh cranberries, coarsely chopped
1 cup raisins or dried cranberries
1/2 cup liquid sweetener (honey works well)
1 t ground ginger
1.5 t red pepper flakes

Mix together all of the ingredients in a small bowl. For best results, make the day ahead and let mellow in the fridge. This can be frozen for later use.

Cucumber

Not only do cucumbers offer a refreshing crunch to salads and dips, they are rich in both nutrients and medicinal properties. Cucumbers offer a fair amount of vitamin C, vitamin A, potassium, manganese, folate, magnesium and dietary fiber. They also contain caffeic acid, which soothes irritated skin.

One of the best uses for cucumbers is not a dietary use, but a cosmetic one. Cucumbers are a valuable source of silica. Silica is an essential mineral in the production of collagen. Internally, they help to improve the complexion, and the high water content is also good for the skin. Cucumbers contain 90% water, which keeps them naturally cooler than their environment. They contain enzymes, which are good at digesting protein and cleansing the body. They are also diuretics.

Externally, cucumbers are soothing to irritated skin. They are also applied to blemishes and inflamed areas, including burns.

As a very low calorie and fat free food, cucumbers are an ideal snack for those wishing to lose weight or balance an otherwise high fat diet. For a salad loaded with fat in other forms, the addition of cucumbers may be just what it needs to become a more balanced meal.

Here's a great way to incorporate the soothing effects of cucumbers into the diet.

Cucumber Raita

1/2 cup organic yogurt
1 T lemon juice
dash salt and pepper
1 cucumber, grated
1 T cilantro
dash dried ginger

Mix all of the ingredients together in a medium bowl. Serve chilled.

Currants

Currants are basically tiny raisins. The tiny champagne grapes native to the Greek isles are dried producing the tangy currant. Many chefs prefer currants to traditional raisins due to their exceptional flavor. Their small size also helps to retain moisture and their shape in baking. Try them in your next batch of oatmeal cookies with this recipe:

Oatmeal Currant Cookies

3 eggs
1 cup currants
1 t pure vanilla
1 cup butter
1.5 cups Sucanat
2.5 cups whole wheat flour
1/2 t salt

1 t cinnamon
2 t baking soda
2 cups oatmeal

Cream together the butter and sugar in a stand mixer. Add the vanilla then the eggs, one at a time. Gradually add the dry ingredients to the mixture. Fold in the currants. Scoop by heaping teaspoonful onto ungreased sheets. Bake at 350 degrees for about 10 minutes.

Dhal

Dhal is a basic Indian food staple. It is technically a refined legume, which makes it easy to cook. You can easily find dhal made from lentils in health food stores, though specialty stores may offer dhal in every legume imaginable. To make dhal, the legume loses its seed coat, then is split in half. When this is cooked with Indian spices, dhal is the result. The nutrient values will represent the values of the legume chosen to make the dish.

Red Lentil Dhal

1.5 cups red lentils
1 t chili powder
1/2 t turmeric
1/2 t salt
2 T ghee
1/2 t cumin seeds
1 T onion salt
2 t dried ginger
1 T lemon juice
dash of salt

Boil the lentils in a pot of water (with 4 cups of water) and the spices (not the seeds) for 30 minutes. Place the ghee in another pot and heat it. Add the cumin seeds and toast them. Add to the soft lentils and serve.

Date

These ancient Middle Eastern foods are actually berries. They are sweet and full of nutrients. As they dry, the sugar content changes from primarily fructose to primarily glucose. This makes them taste sweeter and makes them easier on the liver. The sugar content, being close to 70%, is the primary ingredient, though they also contain iron, niacin and potassium. Dates also provide vitamin A, the B family, selenium and various amino acids, making them a great treat for a dieter with a sweet tooth.

Raw, Vegan Caramel Apples

My friend Sara Janssen (www.WalkSlowlyLiveWildly.com) makes simple raw and vegan caramel apple style snacks by topping an apple slice with a piece of dried date. These are a great way for kids to get some nutrition, but they go quickly, so be sure to chop up plenty of dates and apples!

Oatmeal Date Bars

2 cups pitted dates, chopped well
1 cup organic orange juice
1 t orange zest
2 cups rolled oats
1 cup ground grains (wheat and barley are good choices)
1 t cinnamon
1 t baking powder
1/2 t baking soda
1/2 t salt
1/2 cup liquid sweetener (honey works well)
1/2 cup coconut oil

Combine the dates, juice and zest in a pan. Cook over medium heat until the dates are soft, then remove and set aside. In another bowl, combine the dry ingredients and add the liquid ingredients and the date mixture, mixing well. Press into an 8 inch square pan and bake at 350 degrees for 25 to 30 minutes or until browned.

Eggs

Eggs have suffered through a terrible reputation lately due to their cholesterol content. The good news for eggs is that they also contain a healthy amount of lecithin, which helps the body process cholesterol. The available research does not point to eggs as the source of all elevated cholesterol, which seems to be caused more by unhealthy fats and perhaps some conventional, poor quality eggs. Healthy free range eggs, however, can be a great part of any diet, even for those with elevated cholesterol. The key, as with all foods, is in moderation and a better understanding of the labels on the products. Here's a quick run down of the most common:

Organic eggs: These eggs are from chickens that have been fed organic foods, meeting the organic criteria. They have not been treated with antibiotics or hormones.

Omega 3 enriched eggs: These eggs come from chickens that have been fed diets rich in omega 3 acids. The additional fatty acids can then be found in increased levels in the eggs produced by these chickens.

Brown eggs: Brown eggs are not necessarily any healthier than white eggs. The breed of chicken determines the color of the egg.

Free range eggs: Chickens that have been allowed to move about freely in the fresh air produce these eggs.

Traditional eggs: These eggs come from chickens that have been fed regular feed, are kept in confinement and have not had any special treatment regarding their diet or environment.

As you can see, there is quite a bit of confusion in the types of eggs available and in which eggs are the best to consume. To muddy the waters even further, combinations can also be found. You can get free range brown eggs, or free range omega 3 eggs, and so on. However, the best eggs to consume are fresh, organic or omega 3, free-range eggs from a local farmer.

Like other animal products, eggs need to be cooked for safety and optimal nutrient absorption. Common methods include fried, scrambled and boiled.

Eggs are a great source of protein, selenium, iodine, and vitamin B2. They also contain vitamin B12, phosphorus, vitamin B5 and vitamin D, and are rich in carotenoids including lutein and zeaxanthin.

My favorite recipe for eggs is a great kid friendly one, which makes a quick and easy breakfast. Serve with fresh fruit or a smoothie for a complete meal.

Take a slice of bread (whole wheat sourdough is best) and cut a hole in the middle with a cookie cutter. You can modify the shape to match the season or holiday. (Stars for the 4th of July, hearts for Valentine's Day etc.) In a pan, melt a teaspoon of butter, then place the bread in the warm pan. Crack a whole egg into the hole. Cook over medium heat until the egg is set, then turn the bread over. When fully cooked, remove and serve immediately.

Eggplant

Eggplants are nearly 90% water, making them great for dieters. Potassium is their primary nutritional contribution, but they make a popular vegetarian main dish due to the fact they absorb other contents and flavors well.

Their medicinal values are great, however. In China, they are not recommended for pregnant women as they are clearing to the uterus. These actions, while not ideal for pregnancy, are good for other female complaints, including STDs, cysts, tumors and irregular cycles. Many experts in Chinese medicine suggest eggplant for these common female concerns.

Since eggplant can be bland in taste, it is best served with strong flavors like the feta cheese in this recipe.

Take one large eggplant and cut it into rounds. Toss in 2 t salt and place on paper towels to drain off some of the moisture. Meanwhile, chop 4 cloves of garlic and sauté in 2 T olive oil. Add the eggplant to the plan and sauté until barely tender. Transfer to a baking dish. Top with 8 ounces crumbled feta cheese, 2 T marinated sun dried tomatoes, 1/4 cup fresh basil and 1/4 cup Panko breadcrumbs. Bake at 450 degrees for 3-5 minutes or until hot and the cheese begins to melt. Optional: Serve with pasta sauce for dipping.

Fava Beans

Available only for a few weeks each year, these big flat beans are as historic as they are popular. As other beans, they are a rich source of protein, fiber and iron. They are low in fat, and have no cholesterol.

There is a small group of people, mainly of Mediterranean descent, who have a serious reaction to fava beans. Favism, which is a type of anemia, affects boys who eat the beans or breathe in the pollen.

If fava beans are new to you, try them over pasta in this sauce.

Parmesan Fava Pasta

2 T extra virgin olive oil
1.5 t pureed garlic
1 t dried basil
1.5 cups chicken stock
dash salt and pepper
2 cups cooked fava beans
3/4 pound pasta, cooked
4 oz grated Parmesan cheese

Take 1/2 cup of beans and puree with 2 T of the stock. Set aside. Sauté the garlic with basil in the olive oil. Stir in the chicken stock and bring to a boil with the salt and pepper. Add the pureed beans to thicken the sauce; stir in the cheese. Toss with the cooked pasta and serve with additional grated cheese and a dash of dried basil.

Fennel

This sweet spice is as useful in the kitchen as it is in the medicine cabinet. A member of the Umbellifereae family, fennel is related to celery and parsley. Sweet fennel has a tangy licorice flavor and is used in many herbal remedies.

The main medicinal use of fennel is for digestive purposes. It is a main ingredient in the hundred year old herbal remedy Gripe Water and approved by the German Commission E as a remedy for digestive troubles, especially gas and bloating.

Many also report fennel assists with female complaints and stimulates lactation, though this is a folk remedy, not a proven use.

As a food, fennel contributes vitamin C, fiber, potassium, manganese, and folate. It is packed with antioxidants and anti-inflammatory compounds. Look for fennel in crackers, breads and in Mediterranean cooking.

To add this digestive aid to your diet, try this **free range chicken with figs and fennel**, a popular dish in gourmet restaurants:

1 fennel bulb, chopped in large pieces
8 ounces dried figs, organic and chopped
4-6 free-range chicken breasts
2 T butter
2 medium carrots, cut into 1-inch lengths
1 t fennel seeds, crushed
1 t pureed garlic
1 cup chicken broth
1 cup dry white wine

Rub chicken with salt and pepper. Brown in a pan with the butter, 4-5 minutes per side. Remove chicken from heat. Add the fennel and carrots to the pan and cook until tender, about 3 minutes. Add figs and fennel seeds and cook for an additional 3-4 minutes. Raise the heat to medium high and brown the figs for an additional 2-3 minutes. Add garlic, broth and wine. Cook for 4-5 minutes, then add chicken back to the pan. Reduce heat to medium low and cook an additional 15-20 minutes until chicken is done. Serve with juices over a bed of whole grains.

Figs

Figs are such magical fruits to me. My grandmother had 2 fig trees in her backyard while we were growing up and I always remember having figs (fig preserves) on our morning toast at her house. What a treat! I had no idea all kids didn't get figs for their toast! These Asian / Mediterranean natives are loaded with potassium. Eight ounces of figs yield nearly 30% of your RDA for fiber and 15% of potassium. They are full of manganese and carotenoids like beta carotene and lutein. You can also find phytosterols in figs.

Earning an exotic reputation through mention in the Bible and ancient mythology, these mulberry family members have a unique texture and taste. Sweet, smooth and slightly crunchy, fresh figs are best served with a tangy cheese and a drizzle of honey.

Medicinal properties include aiding digestion and assisting with alleviating constipation. Their leaves are known to reduce the amount of insulin needed by diabetics. In one study, this effect was as simple as adding an extract of fig leaves to the patient's breakfast.

For a simple fig appetizer, try these **honeyed figs with chevre**: Slice a dozen figs in half and arrange in a baking dish. Top with 2 ounces of crumbled chevre, then drizzle with a T of a good vinegar. (Tangy balsamic is a good choice.) Bake at 400 degrees for 5-6 minutes. Serve with a slight drizzle of honey to bring out the sweetness of the figs.

Fish

One of the most common protein dishes has recently become one of the most confusing due to the large pollution that has taken place. In an unpolluted environment, fish can be some of the healthiest foods we consume. Yet, modern day fish requires another look.

Fish, in general, contain high amounts of protein, B vitamins, omega 3 fatty acids and magnesium. Intake of fish has been associated with lower risk of coronary disease, and fish oil supplements are a common treatment for a myriad of disorders.

Nonetheless, fish can be a dangerous source of heavy metals, particularly mercury. Mercury toxicity can cause birth defects, premature aging, vision loss and the onset of certain diseases. The FDA has suggested that children and pregnant or lactating women avoid certain types of fish. The FDA has also set limits on the safety of fish. If the fish contains less than 1 ppm of methyl mercury, it is considered safe. In Canada, however, it has to contain less than 0.5 ppm of methyl mercury to be considered safe. While the lists change from time to time, below is a good guideline on the safety of various types of fish.

Good Choices (little to no mercury)

Wild salmon
Pacific and Atlantic Flounder
Pacific Sole
Sardines
Anchovies
Domestic Shrimp

Farm raised Striped Bass
Rainbow Trout
Tilapia
Other less common fish will fall in this list as well.

Decent Choices (small amounts of mercury)

Mahi Mahi
Atlantic and Pacific Cod
Haddock
Herring
Pacific and Atlantic Halibut
Wild Sea Bass
Wild Grouper
Pollack

Fish to Avoid (high mercury)

Swordfish
Shark
King Mackerel
Chilean Sea Bass
Farm Raised Salmon (Instead, look for Atlantic Salmon or Norwegian Salmon)

These ratings come from the USDA office of seafood. Obviously, the amounts found will vary, and each source will have certain fish cross over between lists from time to time. These are general guidelines. I would also like to see certain people groups added to the list of those that should avoid heavy mercury levels in fish. Any child who has been tested and shown to have high levels of mercury in their body obviously should exercise caution when eating fish that potentially contain mercury. Adults with known mercury build up should also be cautious. Otherwise, the prudent intake of fish can be a healthy addition to the diet.

Pan Seared Sole with Chili Lime Butter

1/2 stick unsalted butter, softened
1 T finely chopped shallot
1 t lime zest

2 t lime juice
1 t red pepper flakes
1/2 t salt

Mix ingredients together and set aside. This is the butter we will use to garnish the fish.

Sprinkle 4 filets with salt. Heat 1 T olive oil in a shallow pan over medium high heat. Two at a time, cook the fish in the heated oil 4-6 minutes until golden, turning halfway through. Remove to a serving dish and garnish with the lime butter and slices of fresh lime if desired.

Flax

Flax is the richest plant source for omega 3s available. With up to 30% oil, flaxseeds strengthen immunity, assist in preventing cancer and help alleviate arthritis. They are also rich in fiber.

The seeds can be purchased and added to baked goods. Look for whole seeds as the high oil content makes them go rancid quickly. The oil can be purchased for adding to smoothies or drinks. It will go rancid quickly, so store it in the fridge and only buy as much as you can consume regularly.

Try adding flax to your diet with these quick and easy kid friendly snacks.

1 cup organic crunchy peanut butter
1 cup sucanat
1 t vanilla
1 cup liquid sweetener (honey works well)
1 cup flaxseed (whole or freshly ground)
4 cups brown rice crisps
1 cup rolled oats

Mix together the peanut butter, sucanat and liquid sweetener. Cook over medium heat for 2-3 minutes until hot. Stir in the remaining ingredients and pour into a greased pan, pressing down. After cooling, cut into bars. Variation: add 1 cup mini chocolate chips to the final step.

Grains

Grains are an entire food group consisting of various members of the grass family. Grains in general are highly nutritious complex carbohydrates. With few exceptions, grains are consumed cooked, not raw, and they can be blended together or with other ingredients beautifully. They contain every nutrient group needed by the body, including protein, carbohydrates, fats, vitamins, minerals, fiber, and plenty of yet to be identified nutrients as well.

A staple of the human diet since the beginning of time, grains have been included in diets from Biblical times and all other ancient societies. They still occupy the largest space on the healthy eating food pyramid.

Grains can be ground and baked, cooked with water to make a moist side dish, incorporated into other dishes such as soups or baked goods or eaten toasted as a finger food. Adding grains to the diet is almost always a healthy idea. Try getting more grains with this **wild and brown rice pilaf** recipe:

4 cups chicken broth
1 cup brown basmati rice
1/2 cup wild rice
1 T butter
1/2 cup diced celery
2 granny smith apples, diced
1/4 cup juice (apple or orange)
2 green scallions, sliced
1/4 cup currants or raisins (optional)
1/2 cup toasted pecans or walnuts
dash salt, pepper, cinnamon and parsley

Cook the rice using the broth as the liquid. (If you have a rice cooker, this is an easy step.) Heat the butter and sauté the celery and apples about 3 minutes. Stir in the rice and all other ingredients, except nuts. Cook about 3-5 minutes until moisture is absorbed, then add the nuts. Serve immediately.

Grapes

This vine bearing fruit is known primarily for the juice it produces. Native to the Middle Eastern and Mediterranean area, grapes are round berries, which naturally yield themselves to a fermented drink cherished by societies and religious ceremonies throughout the years. Dried, they produce raisins, a common childhood snack and additive to cookies and baked goods.

Grapes contribute manganese, vitamin C, vitamin B1, and potassium to the diet. They are also loaded with carotenoids, including alpha carotene, beta carotene, and lutein. They are low in calories and contribute to heart health, thanks to the phytonutrients found in darker colored grapes.

Like most foods, they are best consumed raw. Chilled grapes are a favorite snack of children and frozen grapes can often be passed off as candy to both children and adults alike!

Mediterranean cooking often features grape leaves as well, as a wrap for other dishes. These can be found in health food or gourmet stores. Popular stuffings include rice, meat, lentils and seasonings.

Free range chicken with grapes

4 free range chicken breasts
1/2 cup dry white wine
1/2 cup green grapes

Soak chicken breasts in half of the wine and a dash of salt and pepper. Remove and pan sear over medium high heat with a tablespoon of melted butter. Cook 5-7 minutes each side or until chicken is done. Remove onto a serving dish.

Meanwhile, slice the grapes in half and soak in the remaining wine. Cook grape mixture over medium heat until reduced by half. Add a dash of pepper to the sauce and pour over cooked chicken. Garnish with whole grapes.

Grapefruit

This large citrus food is a perfect source of vitamin C. One half a fruit contains nearly 80% of the RDA. It also offers fiber, potassium, vitamin A, folate, vitamin B5, and multiple carotenoids including both alpha and beta carotene, lycopene and lutein.

Grapefruit is unrelated to table grapes; they get their name because of the way they grow on the vine. They can be found in pink, ruby red and even white varieties. Obviously, the carotenoids are more available in the darker colored selections.

Grapefruit interacts with many pharmaceutical drugs. Some drugs, such as immunosuppressant, calcium blocker, and statin drugs typically require that grapefruit juice be avoided. Other drugs, such as certain antivirals and antihistamines are enhanced with grapefruit. The juice especially makes the drugs more bioavailable to the body. (Note: This should be taken into consideration, as it is a potential risk, not a benefit.)

Lemon Grapefruit Tart

You will need 6-8 personal sized tart shells, which can be found in the freezer section, or you can make your own. In a bowl, mix together 1 diced grapefruit with 1 cup of lemon curd. Scoop into the prepared shells. Top with toasted almonds and grapefruit slices. Serve chilled.

Green Beans

Also known as haricot verts or snap beans, green beans are a nutritional powerhouse. Their boastings include vitamin K, vitamin C, manganese, vitamin A, fiber, folate, iron, potassium, magnesium, vitamins B2, B3 and B1, calcium, phosphorus, protein, carotenoids and even omega 3 fatty acids.

With such a mild flavor, most kids will readily add them to their diets, and the serving possibilities are endless. Try them lightly drizzled with olive oil with a dash of coarse salt then baked at 400 degrees until crisp but done. Or, try them with pine nuts and basil.

Green Beans with Pine Nuts and Basil

Take 1-2 pounds of green beans. Cook them in a pot of boiling water until tender (about 4-6 minutes). Drain and set aside. Meanwhile, heat 1 T olive oil over medium high heat and sauté 1/4 cup pine nuts and 1 t pureed garlic until brown. Add the cooked beans and cook another 4-5 minutes. Top with a handful of fresh basil leaves and a handful of grated hard cheese. Season with salt and pepper.

Grits

I will never forget the time my husband and I played a trivia game with some family members. One relative was given a multiple choice question, "What are grits?" The wrong answer? Potatoes! The right answer? Corn. Grits are as simple as dried corn ground too thick to be cornmeal. The Italian dish polenta features the same ground corn, but with an entirely different serving style.

Grits are typically cooked into a mush then served with butter or cheese. Polenta is cooked, allowed to set, then sliced and cooked again to be topped with pasta sauce or cheese.

Grits contain the same nutritional benefits as corn, since they consist of ground corn. The toppings added will generally make grits more fattening, but that could be a good thing especially in the case of picky eaters.

For traditional grits, try this classic breakfast recipe. Boil 4 cups of water. Add 1 cup yellow stone ground grits and 2 T butter. Cover and cook 15 minutes, stirring well. Remove from heat and let sit 4-5 minutes, still covered while they finish cooking. Serve with salt and more butter.

For an upscale side dish, try these baked cheese grits, a Southern classic.

1 cup milk
3 cups water
1-2 t salt
1 cup yellow grits
dash black pepper
4 T unsalted butter
4 ounces sharp cheddar, shredded

Bring liquid and salt to a boil. Add grits, lower heat and cook, covered for 15 minutes, stirring well. Remove from heat and stir in the rest of the ingredients. Optional: pour into a baking dish and bake at 400 degrees until the top is crisp.

Guava

Guava is an exotic tropical fruit with a deep floral aroma. It is rich in vitamin C, folate, carotenoids, potassium, fiber, calcium and iron. Guava is a mild laxative and slightly astringent.

It can be consumed raw, as a topping on ice cream or desserts. It also makes a welcome addition to a breakfast fruit bar or fruit salad. The pear shaped fruit is typically grown in tropical locations and imported to the mainland.

Try guavas in this breakfast smoothie: Take a banana, guava, mango, handful of strawberries, peach, and other berries and toss into a blender. Add 1/4 – 1/2 cup orange juice and blend until well combined. For an icy treat, use frozen berries. Serve immediately.

Hazelnuts (Filberts)

This nut is a favorite of Europeans, and personally, I agree with them. The toasty flavor has been said to resemble butter and the smooth taste adds to that reputation. There is nothing better than hazelnuts mixed with chocolate, though they also perk up salads and stuffings.

When compared to other nuts, hazelnuts are second only to almonds in calcium content. They also offer protein, iron, fiber, folate and manganese. For a complete list of common nuts and their nutritional value, go to www.hazelnutcouncil.org and click on health analysis.

The FDA has approved a claim that 1.5 ounces of hazelnuts daily reduce the risk of cardiovascular disease. This is important because it is the first such claim allowed for any nut. They are low in saturated fat and cholesterol. Like other nuts, they are a valuable source of high quality fats and proteins.

Since hazelnuts and chocolate mix together to create such decadent treats, this recipe is one of indulgence more than health.

Hazelnut Chocolate Truffles

1 cup toasted chopped hazelnuts
8 ounces organic semisweet chocolate
1/2 cup heavy cream
1 t vanilla extract

Chop the chocolate and place it in a medium bowl. Heat the cream over medium heat until it begins to boil. Immediately pour over the chopped chocolate. Stir together the cream and chocolate. Stir in the vanilla and chill until slightly firm (about 45 minutes). Scoop into 1/2 inch chunks and place on a cookie sheet. Chill another 15-20 minutes. Roll the chunks into balls then roll in the hazelnuts. Place back into the fridge to chill another hour or two.

Honey

Honey is the valuable nectar produced by bees over the course of their lives. Like sugar, it is quickly absorbed and can create hypoglycemic symptoms. Unlike sugar, honey contains valuable enzymes and minerals to aid in its own digestion. The darker the honey, the more mineral rich it is and the stronger taste it has. When heated, many of the nutrients found in honey are destroyed, so most experts prefer raw honey. Honey can also contain a specific form of botulism, which can be fatal in infants. Babies younger than two years should never be given honey.

Local honey is said to help with seasonal allergies. Honey is also a mild laxative and soothes digestion. Try is in herbal teas, as a drizzle for breads or pastries or in baking. For each cup of sugar in baking, substitute 2/3 cup honey and reduce the liquid by 1/4 cup. The baking temperature should be reduced by 25 degrees since honey can cause baked goods to brown faster. Like all sweeteners, it should be consumed in moderation.

Honey Glazed Brie

1/4 cup honey
1 t vanilla extract
1/4 cup toasted pecans
1 medium size brie round

Mix together the honey, vanilla and pecans. Drizzle over the top of the cheese and bake at 500 degrees for 6 minutes. Serve with crusty bread and fresh fruits.

Jicama (Yambean)

This Central American root vegetable is pronounced HEE-kuh-muh. It resembles a turnip, yet when the skin is removed a sweet, crunchy interior is revealed. It is low in sodium and high in potassium. It is also a good source of fiber, iron, omega 3s, folate, and one serving contains 40% of the RDA for vitamin C.

Though it is a vegetable, it is sweet enough to blend in with fruit salads. Toss diced jicama into your next fruit salad to add a bit of crunch. It can be cooked, but will lose much of its flavor.

To truly experience jicama, try it in this Central American dish, **picarda**. Take one jicama, peel it and chop into matchsticks. Squeeze the juice of 3 limes over the vegetable. Mince 3 Serrano chilies and 8 fresh mint leaves. Add to the jicama and lime mixture. Mix well and serve on crisp lettuce leaves.

Kale

This large curly green vegetable is a nutrient powerhouse. One cup of cooked kale contains over 1,300% of the RDA for vitamin K and nearly 200% of the RDA for vitamin A. It also provides vitamin C, manganese, fiber, calcium, potassium, magnesium, folate, vitamin B6, B2 and B1, iron, protein and phosphorus. That same serving will also provide over 10,000 mcg of beta carotene and over 23,000 mcg of lutein, making it great at supporting eye health.

The immunity supporting nutrients found in kale make it a good year round food to include in the diet. It is sweet and hardy, resilient in both cold and hot climates.

Bow Ties with Kale and Chevre

1/2 pound farfalle pasta, cooked
1 T olive oil
1 cup chopped kale
1 cup chopped peppers (your choice, bell work well)
1 T pureed garlic
1/4 cup fresh basil leaves
dash salt and pepper
8 ounces crumbled chevre

In a saucepan, heat the oil and sauté the peppers. Add the garlic and kale, and cook for 5 minutes. Mix with the pasta. Serve immediately, sprinkled with cheese and fresh basil sprigs.

Kamut

Kamut, which means "wheat" in Egyptian is an heirloom Egyptian wheat, about twice the size of our modern wheat. This versatile grain packs a nutritional punch and can even be tolerated by some who are allergic to regular wheat. Legends abound on the origins of this grain, including one outlandish story of a final grain being rescued and grown from King Tut's tomb. While the exact origins are unknown, so is the exact classification, but most experts will put kamut in the durum wheat class.

The nutritional profile is similar to wheat, but with 30% more protein as well as more magnesium, zinc, B vitamins and fatty acids. Though it contains more protein than wheat, the protein is not in the form of gluten; kamut is actually fairly low in gluten.

The flour, assumed to be durum, is ideal for pasta, but it is also useful in other baked goods as well. Try it in this traditional Middle Eastern flatbread.

Ancient Flatbread

2 cups kamut flour
1/2 t salt
1 T honey
2 t baking powder
1 cup yogurt
2 T olive oil

Mix the dry ingredients together and make a well in the middle. Slowly add the wet ingredients, mixing slowly until incorporated. Divide in half and press each half into a round disc no more than 1/2 inch tall. Bake at 400 degrees 8-10 minutes. Cut into wedges and serve with hummus or other fillings / dips.

Kiwi

This tropical fruit is also a delicacy known as Chinese gooseberries. Their bright green interior is loaded with vitamin C. One small fruit will give almost all of the RDA for that vitamin. They also offer fiber, potassium, magnesium, carotenoids and flavonoids. Not only do they offer more vitamin C than an orange, they offer powerful antioxidant protection, and contain a mere 46 calories, making them perfect for dieters.

They are moisture laden fruits, contributing to healthy digestion. An old Chinese remedy for kidney stones is to drink kiwi juice and the Rutgers University Research Department. labeled kiwi as one of the most nutrient dense of our common foods.

They are best consumed raw, as in this **summer salsa**.

3 chopped kiwis
3/4 cup chopped mango
1 T finely chopped chilies
2 T lime juice
2 t honey
3 T cilantro
dash salt and pepper

Mix all ingredients together in a bowl. Serve chilled with fresh corn chips or over a chicken entrée.

Kumquat

These tart little fruits have been called the sour candy of citrus fruits. With a sweet outside and a blast of tart juice inside, they do sound more like a new product for children than a healthy fruit. These mini fruits are the size and shape of an olive, but look like tiny oranges. They are eaten raw and whole, skin and all.

A traditional Chinese remedy for deep colds is a tea brewed with fresh sliced kumquats and fresh ginger. Infuse the two in boiling water and drink it while it is hot.

The best way to enjoy these little fruits is on a fruit and cheese tray with a variety of options for paring. When cooked, however their flavor is released, making them a strong addition to sauces and fruit preserves. Try them fresh and whole, or in this marmalade recipe:

Kumquat Marmalade

4 dozen kumquats, sliced
4 oranges, quartered
6 cups sucanat
juice of 3 large lemons

Soak the chopped fruits in a pot of water. The typical ratio is 3 cups for each cup of chopped fruit. Bring to a boil, then reduce heat. Simmer for 25-30 minutes. Add the sucanat and lemon. Bring back to a boil. This time, cook until 220 degrees is reached. Remove from heat and scoop into prepared canning jars. Seal and store.

Leeks

Leeks are members of the Allium family, making them relatives of garlic and onions. This family plays a valuable role in our health, providing sulfur-containing phytonutrients and reducing the risk of arteriosclerosis and heart disease. They are rich in manganese, vitamin C, iron, folate, and vitamin B6. They are milder than their cousins, making them a good choice for children or those with sensitive digestive tracts. Many consider them to be overgrown scallions, as their flavor and uses are somewhat similar. Leeks however, due to their size, can create a dish all their own, like this simple oven roasted leeks side.

Oven Roasted Leeks

12 leeks
2 T olive oil
1/4 cup walnuts
dash salt and pepper

Trim leeks and cut in half (lengthwise). Place on a baking dish. Top with oil, salt, pepper and walnuts and bake at 400 degrees for 20-30 minutes.

Lemon

Aside from salt and pepper, lemons are one of the world's most popular flavorings. In addition to the tang they contribute to dishes, they also promote healthy digestion, alkalize the body and treat colds and coughs. Rich in vitamin C, potassium and magnesium, lemons are a good source of a few easy minerals. They can be used in everything from appetizers to entrees to desserts and of course, drinks. Soak a classic pound cake with lemon and watch it turn into a gourmet treat, especially when a few berries are tossed on top. Scoop a lemon sorbet into empty lemon rinds for a classic dessert, or make simple tarts with puffed pastry, fresh berries and some lemon curd. Here's the recipe.

Lemon Curd

5 free range omega 3 egg yolks
1 cup dehydrated cane juice
zest and juice of 5 lemons
1 stick butter, diced

Heat water in the bottom of a double boiler. In the top, combine the egg yolks and sugar. Blend thoroughly. Add the lemon juice and zest and place the top over the simmering water below. Whisk as it cooks for about 10 minutes. You want the mixture to coat the back of a spoon but not clump. When it does, remove it from the heat and add the tiny cubes of butter. Let it sit as they melt then stir the mixture together. Place in a medium bowl and chill.

Bake empty mini pie tarts or pastry shells. Let cool then fill with 2 T lemon curd. Top with 2-3 fresh berries and serve chilled.

Lentils

Lentils date back to Genesis when Esau sold his birthright to Jacob for a bowlful of lentil stew. Thousands of years later, lentils are still a nutritional staple, though still not worthy of a birthright. Mild diuretics, lentils also help control blood pressure, cholesterol and balance blood sugar. They are loaded with protein and offer folate, calcium, potassium, magnesium, sodium and vitamin A.

While we typically see the traditional brown lentils, they also come in green, red, and yellow. They are packed with phytonutrients and offer antioxidant protection. Toss a few in your next batch of soup to get a protein and mineral boost, plus a rich mellow flavor.

Moroccan Lentil Soup

2 chopped onions
1 t pureed garlic
1 cup red lentils
1 pound cooked chickpeas
1 15 ounce can diced tomatoes
1 cup sliced carrots
1/2 cup chopped celery
1.5 t ground cardamom
1/2 t cayenne pepper
1/2 t cumin

Add all the ingredients to a large stockpot and simmer for 2 hours with 5 cups of water. Add up to 1.5 more cups of water, if needed. Serve hot with bread.

Lettuce

Lettuce is actually an entire group of foods. Green lettuce, the basis of salads can refer to romaine, butterhead, and so many more. Lettuces in general are good sources of fiber and iron. The darker the green, the more minerals and nutrients. They also contain valuable chlorophyll, vitamins A, K, B1, B2, and C, chromium, and omega 3s.

Low in calories, lettuce is the classic dieting food. Pile a base of lettuces on a plate and top with an assortment of fruits and vegetables for a quick and nutritious dinner anytime. Try this **summertime salad**, and feel free to substitute any foods you have on hand to create your own masterpiece.

5 cups baby greens
1/4 cup dried cranberries
2 diced granny smith apples
4 stalks celery, diced
fresh plump blackberries

3 roma tomatoes, quartered
1/4 cup homemade croutons (recipe follows)
1/4 cup pecans
1/4 cup bleu cheese
honey mustard vinaigrette
homemade croutons:

Take 3-4 slices of bread. Brush bread with olive oil. Sprinkle with salt and pepper. Cut into 1 inch squares or cut into shapes with mini cookie cutters. Bake at 400 degrees for 3-5 minutes or until dried but not brown and crisp. Serve over salads or store in an airtight container for up to a week.

For flavored croutons, add one of the following with the salt and pepper: Dash garlic powder / Italian herbs / Onion powder

Lima Beans

Lima beans are native to Peru, and the smaller ones are also referred to as butter beans. They are great at alkalizing the body and have less fat than other beans, making them ideal for those that are trying to limit fat consumption.

These beans contain molybdenum, fiber, manganese, folate, protein, potassium, iron and magnesium.

Try them in this **Spanish Paella**

3T olive oil
1 pound free range chicken, cubed
1/4 cup chopped onion
1 diced green pepper
1 T pureed garlic
1 t dried thyme
2 cups Arborio rice (also called risotto)
1 cup chopped tomatoes
3 cups chicken broth mixed with 2 cups water
1 cup lima beans
1/2 cup chopped roasted red peppers
1/4 cup chopped parsley

Cook the chicken in the oil until lightly browned. Remove and add onions, garlic, peppers, and thyme. Sauté 2-3 minutes. Add the rice and sauté another minute until the rice becomes transparent. Stir in the tomatoes, broth and water. Bring to a boil and cook for 15 minutes. Add chicken and beans. Stir frequently while cooking for another 10 minutes. Remove from heat and let stand, covered for 5 minutes for flavors to mellow. Top with parsley and serve.

Limes

Another citrus gem, the lime, tends to bring to mind a summery day in Florida, perhaps because of its famous dessert featuring tiny Key Limes. This bright green tropical fruit is tart and tangy, with less acid then lemons, but offers a stronger support for the liver. They can be substituted for lemons in any recipe. I like to substitute half of the lemons for limes to give a rounded citrus flavor. Lime-Lemonade is a popular summery treat in my house.

Limes tend to spice up any dish they are in. Try them in this tart yet spicy dressing.

1 can of chipotle chilies (reserve 1 T sauce)
1 t pureed garlic
3 T lime juice
3 T vinegar
1/4 cup olive oil

If the peppers are not minced, finely chop them, then add the remaining ingredients. Whisk well until combined. Add a dash of salt and pepper.

Macadamia Nuts

These buttery, yet sweet nuts became famous in a simple cookie. They are tender tropical nuts with a smooth mellow flavor. These nuts contain more fat than almost every other vegetarian food. One pound of these nuts contains over 3,500 calories. The fats are healthy fats, however, and Macadamia nuts also offer protein and fiber. Since they are a bit of an indulgence, try them out in this fish recipe:

1 cup chopped macadamia nuts
1/2 cup Panko breadcrumbs
1/4 cup butter
4 fish fillets

Mix together the nuts, breadcrumbs and butter. Bake the fish in a 400 degree oven for 5-7 minutes. Remove and dredge in the nut mixture. Press to coat fully. Return to the oven and bake an additional 8-10 minutes until fish is tender and coating is lightly browned. Serve with a creamy risotto or other rice dish.

Mandarin

Also called tangerines, mandarins are great at alkalizing the body. The name also encompasses clementines and satsumas. Like other citrus, they are rich in vitamin C, fiber, potassium, magnesium, folate, B vitamins and phytonutrients. Mandarins make great salad toppings, and blend well with other fruits as in this recipe.

Pomegranate Chicken with Mandarin

4 free range chicken breasts
2 mandarins, chopped
juice of 3 mandarins
1/4 cup pomegranate juice
1 T each butter and flour

Grill the chicken on an outdoor grill. Sprinkle with salt and pepper prior to grilling if desired. Take the mandarins, both fruit juices, butter and flour and mix together on the stovetop to make a smooth sauce. Add salt and pepper if desired. Spoon over grilled chicken and garnish with mandarin wedges.

Mango

This tropical fruit is actually related to the cashew and is a cooling and refreshing food. Mangoes are rich in vitamin A, C and potassium. They also contain magnesium, B vitamins, copper and a touch of calcium. They make a great addition to any meal, with a wedge on the side to compliment the dish. Mangoes especially compliment desserts and make a great topping for ice cream.

Mango Pilaf

2 cups basmati rice
1 t red pepper flakes
2 t salt
dash pepper
2 cups grated coconut
2 mangoes, chopped
3 T butter
1 T Dijon mustard

Cook rice according to directions. About 5 minutes prior to the finish time, add the remaining ingredients. Serve with grilled chicken and fresh mango wedges.

Maple Sugar and Syrup

Maple syrup is gathered from the maple tree. When dried, it becomes maple sugar, which can be used in place of white sugar in recipes. Approximately forty gallons of sap are reduced to make one gallon of maple syrup. Maple syrup is a healthier choice than white sugar as it contains less sucrose. It still is processed quickly like other sugars, so it should be consumed in moderation. One caution with maple syrup is the lead seams in the metal cans some producers store the syrup in. Canadian maple syrup and certified organic syrup can be considered safe and lead free.

In addition to desserts, maple syrup can add a sweet glaze to vegetables or even main dishes, like in this **Dijon Maple Glazed Salmon**.

4 wild salmon filets
1/2 cup organic butter
1/2 cup maple syrup
1/4 cup Dijon mustard

Mix the mustard, butter and syrup together. Brush the salmon with this glaze while cooking over high heat until flaky and tender.

Margarine

Margarine has been up and down on the healthy foods list over the years. Originally considered a cheap replacement for butter, margarine got a boost when the over consumption of butter was shown to have negative effects. Now that trans-fats are known culprits, margarine is back on the naughty list where it belongs. Certain brands have tried to produce a healthier margarine spread, even designing studies to show health benefits. The best I can say about margarine is that it is neither a real food nor a whole food. While some brands may not appear to adversely affect health now, I have to wonder if they will stand the test of time. My personal opinion is that margarine is a food to be avoided in favor of responsible use of butter, a real food. For this reason, there is not a margarine recipe.

Mate

Yerba Mate (pronounced "yerba mahtay") traditionally refers to a container for brewing tea, but has now come to refer to the tea itself. This South American tea is popular as a coffee substitute since it is only mildly caffeinated. It is a diuretic, and can reduce fatigue and hunger pangs. It has a mild flavor, but due to the caffeine, it may not be tolerated well at night.

Melons

Melon is an entire group of foods including cantaloupe, honeydew, the classic watermelon, and others. They are nearly 95% water, which earns them the thirst quenching reputation we associate with hot, summery days. They are not typically cooked, and can aid digestion when consumed with a meal.

Considering these properties, melons lend themselves nicely to an appetizer. Try this sweet and tangy treat.

Bleu Cheese Melon Appetizer

Mix together 8 ounces bleu cheese with 8 ounces cream cheese. Take a small, firm melon and remove the insides. Fill with the cheese blend. Serve with assorted melon balls, other fruits and crackers.

Mesclun

Mesclun is the French term given to a blend of young baby lettuces. Mesclun also often includes herbs and edible flower blossoms. These salad blends are readily available and should be used soon after purchase. Not only do they offer an assortment of nutrients found in the greens contained within, they make a pleasing display and a nice base for a colorful salad.

Milk

When the ancient Israelites were promised a land flowing with milk and honey, the image of our modern homogenized and ultra pasteurized white liquid in a jug was not what went through their minds. Milk is a misunderstood food group in and of itself, one that entire books can be written about, yet I will attempt to make sense of the hodge-podge of information in this brief space.

When most people typically think of milk, they think of white jugs in the store with ultra pasteurized, homogenized cow milk with an expiration date stamped on top. This method "improves" the milk, making it safer and more pleasant to drink. Let's look at what exactly we do to milk and see if we really need or want these improvements.

Homogenization - Verb : to prepare an emulsion, as by reducing the size of the fat globules in (milk or cream) in order to distribute them equally throughout

Remember your grandmother telling you about skimming the cream off the milk? If you grew up on a farm, you may remember the cream separating from the milk and being stirred back in. Apparently, that is an undesirable cosmetic characteristic of milk. Homogenization takes this layer of fat and reduces the size of the fat particles, making it disperse into the milk, so separation does not take place. Unfortunately, the size of a fat particle plays an important role in its digestion. The smaller fat globules can fit through places that they really have no business fitting through. Many experts believe this leads to heart disease. Goat milk is naturally homogenized, but cow milk homogenization is an artificial process. It is not difficult to find milk that is not homogenized in most areas. Milk can be pasteurized without being homogenized.

Pasteurization - Verb: The process of heating a liquid for the purpose of destroying harmful organisms, named after the French scientist, Louis Pasteur.

The pasteurization process is one that is heavily debated among health professionals. Some would argue that without it, milk would be virtually toxic due to all the harmful microbes found inside it. Others will argue that a cautious farmer with well cared for cattle (or goats) can produce healthy raw milk, perfectly suitable for human consumption. These same enthusiasts will argue that the heating of the milk kills off healthy enzymes and beneficial organisms along with the bad, and the shelf life is greatly reduced. I have to argue that both sides make a very valid point. In certain cases, especially with negligent farmers, raw milk can be dangerous. Some US states certify raw milk, which means they have an inspection process and raw milk is legally sold for human consumption. In other states, however, raw milk is not legally sold for human consumption.

I agree that the benefits of raw milk are many, but in states with no legal recourse in the event of bad farming practices, raw milk may pose a danger. Either way, I never recommend pregnant or nursing mommies, children under the age of five, and any elderly individuals consume raw milk, and I suggest strong caution in areas that do not certify raw milk.

This is not to assume that certification is a guarantee of safety, yet the simple fact that the buyer has recourse in the event of careless activity provides some motivation for the farmer to maintain high standards. Cheese and other dairy products made from raw milk can be purchased in just about every health food store.

The unfortunate fact about milk is that most people tend to consider the product as making up an entire food group of its own. No other mammal consumes the milk of another animal. I do not consider drinking milk to be a bad practice, but I do question the emphasis we place on consuming this one product. While milk can play a role in good health, it is not required.

Milk alternatives also exist. Goat milk is nutritionally superior to cow milk, especially for children. Not only is it higher in fat, it contains far more calcium, vitamin A, B6, potassium, selenium and niacin. In fact, only 2 nutrients are more plentiful in cow milk than goat milk, and these are only slight differences. The proteins in goat milk, being somewhat similar to human milk, are much easier to digest than cow milk, making it better for children who often have difficulty with cow milk. Many people who are allergic or sensitive to cow milk can tolerate goat milk.

Milk is also available in healthier forms than liquid. The processes of making cheese, kefir, and yogurt all aid in the partial digestion of the proteins in milk, making nutrients available, digestion easier, and adding probiotics to the food.

Millet

Millet is a tiny (seed) grain that is packed with nutrients. One serving of millet can offer nearly a third of the RDA for manganese and magnesium. It also offers plenty of phosphorus. Millet is useful in prevention of type 2 diabetes, preventing heart disease, repairing body tissues and preventing kidney stones. Millet does contain goitrogens, which are substances that can inhibit the use of iodine, adversely affecting thyroid function, so those with thyroid problems should avoid consuming it.

Millet can be ground into a flour and used in place of some of the wheat flour in a muffin or quick bread recipe. It can be cooked into a fluffy comfort food or a thick risotto style dish. When cooked, it is quite similar to rice, so the possibilities are numerous. My children enjoy it in the morning in the breakfast cereal recipe below.

Apple Millet

Bring 2.5 cups of apple juice to a boil. Add 1 cup of millet and 1 t salt. Simmer for about 20 minutes or until all the juice is absorbed. Fluff with a fork and serve with cinnamon and butter and / or maple syrup.

Molasses (treacle)

Molasses is an old fashioned sweetener, with many stories to tell. The term "slow as molasses" is a common one, but once in history, molasses was not that slow. In 1919, during the height of the popularity of molasses, a molasses tank in Boston exploded, sending the sweetener flowing through the streets. Two point three million gallons of molasses went spewing through the streets forming thirty foot waves and crushing everything in its path. It knocked over a fire station, crumpled the steel support of a train bridge and killed 21 people, while injuring 150 others.

More practically, molasses is the thick, dark sweetener left over from the processing of sugar. It has a mild laxative effect, and blackstrap molasses, which comes from the third boiling in the process, is rich in minerals as well. The first two boilings produce lighter molasses, with a higher sugar content. Conversely, blackstrap molasses has a higher concentration of nutrients but lower sugar content, making it an ideal healthy sweetener. While blackstrap molasses appears to be an amazing food, I feel the need to caution against the use of any non-organic blackstrap molasses. As a concentrated source of nutrients, it is great, but, by concentrating the compounds within the sugar, it also creates a concentration of the toxins as well. This should not be a problem with organic blackstrap molasses, which would not have the pesticide residues and other indirect additives. Additionally, sulfur is often used in processing, so unsulfured organic blackstrap molasses is the way to go.

The nutrients found in blackstrap molasses include manganese, copper, iron, calcium, potassium, magnesium, vitamin B6, and selenium - quite an impressive. nutritional profile for a sweetener!

With the exception of gingerbread cookie baking during the holidays, Americans don't use much molasses anymore. Despite the nutritional benefits, molasses has a strong flavor that leaves a distinct mark among the treats it sweetens. This makes it ideal for ginger cookies and gingerbread during the holidays, but I also like to use it in a homemade granola recipe:

Molasses Sweetened Granola

6 cups oats
2 cups blackstrap molasses
1 cup brown rice syrup
2 cups pecans
1/2 cup coconut oil
3 cups brown rice crisps
2 T vanilla
1 t cinnamon

1 t salt
1 cup dried cranberries

Mix all ingredients together in a large bowl. Press into a greased 9x13 inch baking pan. Bake at 350 degrees for 30 minutes. Remove and cool before cutting into bars. This large batch can be cut in half easily with great results.

Alternate recipe: omit the cinnamon, pecans and cranberries. Substitute 1 cup chunky peanut butter for the 1/2 cup coconut oil and add 2 cups chocolate chips. Bake as directed.

Mushrooms

Mushrooms are actually an entire family of fungal fruits. These little fungi have a respectable reputation as a health food for good reason. They are rich in phytonutrients, which help us detoxify our bodies. They offer selenium, vitamins B2, B3, B5, B1 and B6, copper, potassium, phosphorus, zinc, manganese, protein, folate, fiber, magnesium, calcium and iron. Mushrooms are also known to boost the immune system and even increase longevity, which may be why the ancient Romans considered them to be a "food of the gods," and the Egyptians thought they were magical.

Mushrooms are also a rich source of glutamic acid, which plays a key role in the umami factor. In more practical terms, this simple means they enhance the flavor of foods with which they are cooked.

Since wild mushrooms can be toxic, it is best to only consume identified mushrooms. Most store bought mushrooms are cultivated, and the identity can be certain. Some of the healthiest varieties are crimini mushrooms, and their overgrown version, portabella mushrooms. These mushrooms have an abundance of antioxidants. Shitakes are also healthy mushrooms, used in many countries to boost the immune system and fight cancer.

Stuffed Mushrooms

24 Crimini mushrooms, boiled for 3 minutes and stems removed
1/2 cup Panko breadcrumbs
1/2 cup hard cheese
2 T Italian seasoning
1 t pureed garlic

2 T olive oil

Mix together all of the ingredients except for the mushrooms. Stuff the filling in the mushroom cavities. Bake at 375 degrees for 20-30 minutes until browned.

Nori

This seaweed is typically reserved for sushi and other adult gourmet foods, but it actually makes a great addition to many dishes. It contains calcium, iodine, sodium, vitamins A, C, and B complex, protein, potassium and zinc. It also contains valuable cancer fighting properties.

Despite having a reputation as being more appropriate for a mature palate, nori is a great food for kids. The texture makes a perfect finger food for toddlers, and when given the chance, many kids will love sushi. Try this simple, mild tasting recipe to introduce them to sushi, and let them have fun experimenting with various fillings.

Nori Sushi

2 cups sushi rice (stickier in texture than plain rice), cooked
3 T rice vinegar
1 t salt
4-5 sheets nori
assorted fillings including avocado strips, carrot strips, asparagus, jicima, mushrooms, etc.

Combine the rice, salt and vinegar. Lay out one sheet of seaweed and cover it with rice. Add the desired toppings. With a bamboo rolling board, roll the rolls up as tightly as possible. Slice into 1 inch portions. Serve with soy sauce if desired.

Nutritional Yeast

Nutritional yeast is a popular item in health food stores. Though it is not a natural food, it seems to benefit some individuals. It is basically yeast that was grown primarily on molasses, then pasteurized. It offers a variety of nutrients, especially B vitamins. Part of its popularity is gained from the B12 content. While many appreciate its nutritional content, I personally prefer consuming natural, real foods that offer beneficial nutrients.

Oats (Avena Sativa)

This common grain is a classic example of how a nourishing food can easily be widely available. Oats can stand up to many things including drought and harsh soil conditions. Yet, they still offer many protective benefits in addition to their nutritional content.

Oats offer manganese, selenium, phosphorus, B1, protein, magnesium and fiber. They also offer an impressive assortment of carotenoids. Oats are often the only source of whole grains in many diets. In a restaurant, oats will more than likely be the only whole grain choice on the menu.

Medicinally, oats help stabilize the blood sugar, reduce cholesterol, regulate the thyroid, soothe the nervous and digestive systems, and can even be beneficial in weight loss.

Many types of oats are easy to find in any store. Oat groats, also called Scottish oats or Irish oatmeal, are the unflattened kernels, which can be used for stuffing or as a breakfast cereal. Steel cut oats are simply whole oats that have been run through a machine that slices them into 2-3 sections. These cook faster than whole oats and have a slightly chewy texture. Sometimes, steel cut oats are referred to as Scottish oats or Irish oatmeal as well. Old fashioned or rolled oats are whole oats that have been flattened by a machine with 2 big rollers. When they are cut before rolling, they are quick cooking oats. The rolling process itself provides for a faster cooking time than whole oats.

Oats are considered by some professionals to be gluten free, while others list them as low gluten. The difference appears to be an issue of cross contamination, and many people with celiac disease can tolerate them in moderation. Some celiac support groups even list oatmeal as a gluten free food, but many companies process oats on equipment that is shared with wheat, so this is a tough consideration for those with celiac disease or gluten intolerance.

Simple Granola

These yummy toasted oats can be used in so many ways. Try tossing them on top if your next batch of muffins, over ice cream or even in cookies. Keep a little jar of them on the counter and you will find the options are endless.

1 cup old fashioned oats
1 T vanilla
1 T maple syrup

In a saucepan over medium heat, add the oats and cook about a minute, stirring constantly. Slowly begin to pour the vanilla and syrup over the oats. Cook until they are browned and all the flavorings have been absorbed. Remove from heat and let cool. Store in an airtight container.

Okra

This southern summertime vegetable is as versatile as it is healthy. Okra is rich in B vitamins, vitamin C and potassium. The sticky mucilage is useful in cases of constipation, as it soothes an irritated digestive tract. It also serves to thicken soups and stews, which is the main use in culinary preparations in the Deep South, particularly Louisiana. Others however, love to slice it, batter it and fry it, making a crispy little snack or side dish. My personal favorite is to roast the entire pods with a drizzle of olive oil salt and pepper. The resulting slightly crispy is a true summertime treat. Here's how

Take a half a pound of okra. Wash it well, then place on paper towels to drain. Prepare a baking sheet and hot (400 degree) oven. Place the entire okra pods onto the sheet, drizzle with about 2 T olive oil and sprinkle 1-2 t each or coarse salt and freshly ground pepper. Bake for 10-15 minutes or until the okra begins to brown. Serve immediately.

Olives / Olive Oil

Olives, the traditional Mediterranean fare, have made themselves known worldwide as an indispensable culinary ingredient, medicinal tool and even beautifying agent. One of the oldest foods available, mentioned in the Bible and other ancient texts, olives are well deserving of their renowned reputation.

Olives are actually never consumed raw. They contain a bitter glycoside, which makes them inedible. When soaked in brine, pressed into oil or processed in like manner, the glycosides are removed, making them extremely healthy foods. Some olives are soaked in a lye solution to remove the glycosides. This process effectively inhibits the bitterness, but I much prefer the other available methods of preparing olives for consumption.

Whole olives offer healthy amounts of iron, fiber, copper, loads of carotenoids, and plenty of healthy fat. In addition to their heart benefits, they can assist with inflammatory problems such as arthritis and asthma. Research indicates that those consuming a diet rich in olives and their oil are less likely to suffer from rheumatoid arthritis. They can be found green and black, ranging from sour to bitter, all depending on the processing. Gourmet olives tend to be worth their high cost as they offer far more flavor. In my opinion, the best olives are Kalamata, Liguria and Nicoise. These are not soaked in lye, are tree ripened and offer the most nutrients and flavor.

Olives may best be known for their oil, however, namely the extra virgin kind, which comes from the initial pressing of the olives. This oil is roughly 75% oleic acid, which is a heart healthy monounsaturated fat. It also offers protective antioxidants and phytonutrients. Olive oil is one of the primary reasons researchers tend to favor the Mediterranean diet.

Since we live or die at the cellular level, any food that provides powerful antioxidants and promotes cellular health in turn promotes overall health. Monounsaturated fats are more difficult to damage than others, which in turn offers a bit of a protective benefit to the cells. When this is coupled with the antioxidant abilities, it is easy to see how this little food became such a legend.

Olive oil is also used to treat peptic ulcers, which recent research has shown can be caused by *Helicobacter pylori* infections. This is great news, since these have recently begun to be treated with antibiotics and the bacterium has already begun to become resistant to these antibiotics. The olive oil seems to survive the acidic environment of the stomach, and even aid in the strands, which are antibiotic resistant.

It also is used for lowering cholesterol, supporting the liver, balancing blood sugar and as an aid in weight control. While the health benefits are numerous, the only potential drawbacks are for those on a low fat diet. However, when we consume fat, this is one of the best kinds to consume.

Olive oil, like other liquid oils, can become rancid quickly. Aside from the occasional drizzle atop vegetables, olive oil is best consumed at room temperature. Olive oil can be pricey, but with a little research, it can be found with both high quality and an affordable price.

Olive Tapenade

Olive tapenade is a spread made from olives and a few spices. While it is typically served with vegetables or pita wedges, it can also be served atop tomatoes, fish or chicken. Simply take a half a pound of chopped olives and mix them with pureed garlic (1T), 2 T chopped parsley, 1 T lemon juice, salt and pepper, 1 T olive oil, and 1 T Dijon mustard.

Onions

Like garlic, their close cousins, onions are one of the healthiest foods. In addition to their strong flavor, onions provide fiber, vitamin C, vitamin B6, calcium, folate, potassium and a touch of iron and zinc. Their main contribution, however, lies in the stores of carotenoids, flavonoids and phytonutrients found in the bulbs. One of the flavonoids, quercetin, protects against cataracts, heart disease and even cancer. Their sulfur compounds help to lower blood pressure, lower cholesterol and improve kidney function. In addition, onions contain chromium, a difficult to find mineral that helps to regulate blood sugar levels. Not only are onions strong antioxidants, they have antibacterial, anti-inflammatory, and antiviral properties.

Some onions are grown in low sulfur soil, making them far sweeter than standard onions. Many experts believe these are not as healthy as the standard onions because of their high sugar content. Since the sulfur compounds are part of the health benefits, this is understandable. Onions are also known for irritating the eyes while being prepared. Studies indicate that, essentially, the more irritating an onion is, the healthier it is, because these same properties are what also give us many of the health benefits.

Studies also reveals that both onions and garlic are healthier after they have been cut and exposed to air for a few minutes. In fact, recent studies have shown that, even when heated, which was previously thought to destroy the medicinal properties of onions and garlic, these nutrients remain if they have been exposed to air prior to heating. This exposure turns the phytonutrients into health promoting compounds. This can be increased the finer the onion is chopped. The accompanying scent and eye irritation will also increase as the healthy compounds become stronger.

For a nutrient packed entrée, try this **Garlic Parmesan Pasta**, which actually contains both onions and garlic.

Take 1 cup chopped onions (any size / type) and 2 T garlic puree and place in a medium saucepan with 1 T olive oil over medium heat. Sauté 3-4 minutes. Add 1/4 cup dry white wine and 1/4 cup chicken broth (or 1/2 cup broth and omit the wine). Simmer 5 minutes. Add 1/4 cup shredded hard cheese such as Parmesan and stir into the sauce. Immediately add 1/2 pound of cooked pasta with 2 T reserved water from the pasta. Serve with additional cheese on top.

Oranges

Historically, oranges were special occasion items. They were expensive, typically used as gifts for weddings and Christmas. Now, they are readily grown in warm weather states and inexpensive to consume year round. Their compact shape and all inclusive wrapper makes them ideal for snacking on the go, and the high water volume makes this snack as thirst quenching as filling.

Over 60 flavonoids have been found in oranges. Since they work synergistically with vitamin C, which is also abundant in oranges, the health benefits are enormous. These flavonoids are anti-inflammatory, anti-tumor, and have blood clot inhibiting properties. Oranges also offer fiber, folate, thiamin, calcium, vitamin A, and potassium.

Oranges generally taste best raw, which is the best way to obtain the maximum nutrients of most fruits and vegetables. The zest or essential oil can be removed from the peel and is often used as a flavoring for baking. Since the pesticides tend to accumulate on the thick peel, it is best to only bake with organic zest or essential oil. Otherwise, we may be adding a concentrated source of toxins into our baked goods.

The peels also contain a group of compounds called poly-methoxylated flavones. These have the potential to lower cholesterol more effectively than many prescription drugs.

Oranges also offer the popular breakfast juice of the same name. While this is a great source of many of the nutrients, it generally lacks the fiber found in the whole food. Remember that unless the juice is freshly squeezed, many of the nutrients are lost in the processing and transporting to our homes. There are also important nutrients found to lower blood pressure and cholesterol that are in the white pulp, which is often eliminated in the juicing process. Which goes back to one of my main points:, foods are best consumed in their "whole" or natural state.

Strawberry Orange Pops

Try this healthy alternative to popsicles during the warm summer months. Not only will the kids stay hydrated, the sugars are natural, there are no artificial colors, and there is a boost of nutrients as well!

Take 6-8 whole oranges. Peel and chop into cubes. Place in a blender with about 15 whole strawberries. Pulse until just barely liquid with a few large chunks. Add 5-6 more strawberries, chopped, if desired. Pour into freezer molds (or: place in paper cups and insert a popsicle stick) Place in the freezer. Remove and enjoy

Oysters

The name oyster is actually the name of a group of mollusks that grow in marine water. These edible mollusks are quite impressive as they are also the legendary pearl producers. Additionally, there is a species of crabs that can coexist inside the shell. These are pretty rare and thus valued. Since both oysters and crabs lack fins and gills, they are considered unclean animals for those that use the Levitical guidelines.

Palm Oil / Palm Kernel Oil

Both palm oil and palm kernel oil come from the African palm tree. The palm oil is pressed from the fruit, while the palm kernel oil is pressed from the seed (kernel). Regular palm oil is a bright red color and often used in soap making for its emollient properties as well as the bright color it contributes. Palm kernel oil, however, is a faint light brown. Like coconut oil, oils from the African palm are highly saturated. Thus they are also not generally thought of as a good source of fats. Like all oils, the unrefined brands are the best purchase. The fact that the oil is saturated is not necessarily a bad thing. If a solid fat is needed, a naturally saturated fat is far better than a hydrogenated fat.

Palm oil (the bright red one) is a great source of beta carotene. It also offers other nutrients such as vitamin E. Palm kernel oil (the brown one) is used for candy making and other baking that requires a solid fat. The virgin oil, whether palm or palm kernel does not smell as sweet as coconut oil, making the uses limited. The smell can be removed however, expanding the culinary options.

Papayas

These Central American fruits are grown on what Columbus called the "melon tree" because the huge fruits literally grow on a large herb tree. They range from 1-20 pounds, and when ripe, have bright orange flesh. This fruit offers vitamins C, K, A and E, potassium, folate, fiber and a load of carotenoids.

Perhaps the best known benefit of papayas is in the form of enzymes, particularly papain. This enzyme helps to digest protein and is often sold on its own as a dietary supplement. It is also often recommended for allergic reactions, since many reactions are believed to be due to undigested proteins in foods.

Papayas also contain other beneficial enzymes in addition to the famed papain. Chymopapain is an anti-inflammatory, which means it is beneficial in aiding diseases that get worse with inflammation, such as allergies and asthma. It also helps with burns and stomach ulcers.

For a healthy older baby or toddler snack, chop up avocados and papayas into 1 inch cubes. Not only is this soft snack easy for babies to pick up and mash, the combined nutrients value is huge.

For a more naughty treat, blend 1 papaya (seeds removed) with vanilla ice cream (equal parts) and scoop back into the papaya half shell. Serve chilled as a dessert.

Passion Fruit

The Jesuits named the passion fruit, as they felt it resembled the passion of Christ. Each of its parts were symbolic and used to retell the story to those they attempted to convert. We typically only see the juice at the grocer; the Brazilian fruit is far less common.

Passion fruit is loaded with fiber. It offers vitamins A, C, K and several Bs. You can also find calcium, iron, magnesium, potassium, copper, sodium and zinc in this exotic fruit. Researchers at the University of Florida have found that yellow passion fruit extracts can kill cancer cells in vitro. The phytochemicals, which are responsible for this anti-cancer effect, are carotenoids and polyphenols.

This vinaigrette calls for whole fruits but can easily be adjusted to accommodate the juice if that is all that is available in your area.

4 freshly juiced passion fruits (about 1/4 cup juice)
2 T orange juice
2 T fresh lime or lemon juice
(The juice total should be roughly 1/2 cup.)
2 t honey
2 t Dijon mustard
1/2 cup olive oil
salt and pepper to taste

Whisk together until fully combined. Serve over a fresh green salad with plenty of fresh fruits added and some tangy cheeses.

Pasta

Pasta is the term used for a warming starch substance typically made from wheat, especially durum wheat. It can also be made from other flours such as rice, potato and even vegetables. As far as health is concerned, pasta has plenty of potential as a health food, provided quality ingredients are used in preparing the food. Pasta is easy to digest, making it an ideal grain source for those with difficulty digesting bread or other baked goods. Whole wheat pasta contains far more fiber than white pasta, which is typical with all flour products.

Pasta is a highly versatile food. Not only can it be used as a main dish, it makes a perfect side dish. The countless sizes and shapes combined with numerous sauces for pairing make the possibilities literally endless. Many chefs suggest pairing thick and chunky pastas with similar sauces, leaving thin sauces for the thinner pastas, but I personally love to mix and match all around for a variety of flavors and texture of a dish.

One of my favorite pasta dishes combines a simple to find penne with fresh green peas for a light yet filling meal. Serve it with a crusty bread and summer salad.

Penne With Baby Peas and Feta

1 pound penne, cooked
1 cup chicken broth
1/2 cup baby green peas (fresh or frozen)
2 boneless skinless chicken breasts, grilled and sliced into strips
1/4 cup sun dried tomatoes, sliced
1/2 cup feta
1/4 cup Parmesan, grated
spices, as referenced below

Pour a tablespoon of olive oil into a pan over medium heat. Add 2 teaspoons minced garlic and 2 T finely chopped onion. Sauté 2-3 minutes until aromatic. Deglaze with the chicken broth and 2 cups water. Simmer 4-5 minutes until reduced by 1/3. Toss in the cheeses, tomatoes, chicken and pasta. Stir well. Add the peas and cook until tender, about 3 minutes. Serve warm with additional cheese over the top.

Peas

Peas are actually quite the historic food. Consumed for literally thousands of years, they were traditionally eaten dried, not fresh, and were prized by the ancients. The term pea actually refers to multiple vegetables, typically green and round. When consumed freshly picked, their flavors are at a peak, as are the nutrients. In general, peas offer vitamins A, K, C and B complex, as well as calcium fiber, iron, and potassium.

Peas are great bone builders, as not only do they offer calcium, but vitamin K, which leads to optimal bone mineralization. They are also healthy for digestion, and help to strengthen the liver.

Peas can be consumed in numerous ways. The classic split pea soup is an example of a warming nourishing meal, but peas also play a great supporting role as a side dish to just about any entrée. Fresh peas should be featured on their own so the flavor can really stand out.

Perfect baby peas

Boil about 4 cups of water. Add 1 pound of fresh baby green peas and stir continually for about 2 minutes. Remove from heat, drain any extra water and place into a shallow bowl, letting plenty of steam escape. Top with a pat of organic butter and a dash of sea salt.

Peaches

This plum family member is probably one of my favorite fruits. While canned peaches are available year round, the ripe, fresh enticing peach is only available during a short season every summer. I vividly recall my daily trip to the local grocer looking for the fresh peaches I craved throughout my first pregnancy. I literally ate 4-6 of them a day once they ripened!

As it turns out, it was a pretty wise choice. Not only do fresh peaches offer a creamy tart and tangy flavor, but also they are hydrating, which I needed during my summer pregnancy. They also offered this pregnant mommy plenty of nutrients including fiber, calcium, potassium, vitamins A, C, E, and B complex, magnesium and zinc.

While peaches are ideally consumed raw and fresh, they make an even better pie. Try this one, which has been doctored up a bit.

1 cup sucanat
1/3 cup whole wheat flour
1 t cinnamon
4 cups fresh peaches
2 T butter
frozen wheat pie crust (with a "lid")

Combine all the filling ingredients in a medium bowl. Gently stir to coat. Place into the bottom of the crust. Top and crimp the edges. Bake at 400 degrees for 45 minutes.

Peanuts

Peanuts are actually not nuts at all, as any mom of an allergic child will readily tell you. They are legumes, totally unrelated to tree nuts. However, they store fat, not starch, which makes them resemble a nut more than a bean. Nonetheless, since George Washington Carver found over 300 uses for this legume, they have remained an inexpensive staple to many diets, especially children's. However, a survey showed that the incidence of peanut allergy has doubled between 1997 and 2002 among children.

In addition to those with allergies, anyone with cancer, liver problems or Candida should avoid peanuts.

Aside from the caveats, peanuts can boast a great nutritional profile. In addition to healthy fats and proteins, they offer manganese, B complex vitamins, copper, and plenty of phytosterols. They also offer anti-inflammatory properties and plenty of antioxidants.

To obtain the benefits, however, peanuts need to be consumed cooked, not raw. They can be roasted at home, but unless you are getting them from your own garden or directly from the grower, they probably have been previously roasted.

Peanuts should only be purchased organic. One of the best uses for peanuts is as a crop rotator in cotton fields. Since cotton is difficult to grow organically, and since it is not a food crop, stronger chemicals are used on these crops. These fields become laden with harmful chemicals, many of which are not legally used directly on food crops. Studies show us that the chemicals used on these crops are highly stable in the environment and can linger for decades. When the soil is then used to grow peanuts, many of these chemicals are then passed into the food chain and can accumulate in the fatty tissues of both animals and people.

Peanut butter is a common preparation of peanuts, with a great array of fats and protein, but again, it is important to be sure you are getting the real thing. Common peanut butters add sugar and oils to produce the creamy substance of our childhood memories. You will also find a much better fatty profile in almond or cashew butters. Peanut oil is another great use of peanuts, however it is highly difficult to obtain organic oil, which would be void of the harmful chemicals.

The USDA also allows a certain percentage of a mold named aflatoxin (which is a carcinogen), to exist in commercial peanuts. This mold is much more common in the humid southern states than it is in drier ones, and it is a danger worth taking into consideration. To reduce this risk, store peanut products in a dry cool environment.

Peanuts make an easy addition to many meals from main dishes to sides, condiments and even desserts. They pair well with chocolate and form the base of this **classic cookie**.

1 cup peanut butter
1 egg
1/2 cup sucanat
1/2 cup wheat flour

Mix together and form into about 2 dozen balls. Place on an ungreased cookie sheet and bake at 375 degrees for about 10-12 minutes until golden. Remove and set aside to cool. Melt 1/4 cup organic chocolate chips and drizzle over cooled cookies in a zigzag pattern. Once fully cooled, store in an air tight container.

Pears

This autumn fruit is closely related to the apple, but has a texture that has been described as "buttery, yet somewhat grainy." Since they are so close to apples, they also have the same high pectin content, making it great at treating diarrhea and soothing inflamed mucus membranes.

Pears also offer an array of nutrients, including fiber, potassium, vitamin C, copper and vitamin K. They are members of the rose family and come in a variety of colors traditionally associated with their harvest season, red, yellow and brown.

To obtain the best of the laxative and soothing properties of a pear, try grilling them as a side dish or snack.

Cinnamon Grilled Pears

Place 6 halved and cored pears into a bowl of 1/3 cup apple juice to marinate. Add a dash of cinnamon. Place directly onto a hot grill and brush with melted butter. (Make a mixture of 1/4 t cinnamon and 2T butter for brushing.) Cook about 3 minutes on each side, then remove and serve hot.

Pecans

Pecans are another great vegetarian protein source. They are my absolute favorite nuts, as I have vivid memories of gathering pecans from my Grandmother's yard every fall for shelling and baking pies for Thanksgiving. Pecans grow on massive trees, and are the only tree nut native to America.

Pecans are a great source of antioxidants, primarily due to their vitamin E content. This vitamin E helps to protect lipids form oxidation. They contain the highest antioxidant concentration of all nuts. They also contain plant sterols, which have cholesterol lowering abilities. Though they are naturally high in fat, they have been suggested to have the ability to increase the metabolic rate, making them actually ideal for dieting. The fat they do contain is a heart healthy one, making it a healthy addition to the diet.

Pecans can also boast an array of nutrients, including almost 10% of the RDA for fiber (in one ounce), as well as vitamin A, vitamin E, folic acid, calcium, magnesium, phosphorus, potassium, several B vitamins and zinc.

For the dedicated pecan fan, in 2001, April was declared to be the National Pecan Month in the US, thanks to Senator Max Cleland. To celebrate, pecans can easily be added to just about any meal. They make great additions to breakfast fare, snacks, main courses, sides, and even desserts. Just about the only place they don't belong is in the dish of baby food, as most babies should wait until their second birthday to consume nuts, just in case of allergies.

For a protein punch, try this **pecan crusted chicken** recipe. It goes great atop a bed of salad greens or as the entrée for a hearty meal.

1 cup pecans, crushed
1/2 cup wheat bread crumbs
2 eggs
2 pounds chicken cutlets
salt and pepper to taste

Combine the pecans, bread crumbs and salt and pepper in a shallow bowl. In another bowl, whisk the eggs. Dredge the chicken in the eggs then the pecan mixture, making sure it is evenly coated. Place in a baking dish and bake at 375 degrees for 20-30 minutes until evenly browned.

Peppers

Peppers were once the most important spice in world trading. In fact, the money from this trade is what made America's first millionaire. Peppercorns are a stimulant, digestive aid, and have anti-inflammatory effects. It is important to note that peppercorns and peppers are not related.

When we look at peppers, we begin talking about an entire variety of foods. Generally, these peppers fall into two categories, chile and sweet. Chile peppers contain a chemical called capsaicin, which is used in herbal medicine and gives them their kick. Sweet peppers do not contain this chemical, making them more like a vegetable, milder and useful for dishes for a milder palate.

Chile peppers, which were covered earlier in this chapter, are often used for spicy foods, such as salsas, and other ethnic dishes. Sweet peppers find their way into stir fries, sandwiches and are even stuffed with rice and meat, serving as a flavorful bowl. Since I tend to like a little zing in my dishes, I am including a homemade salsa recipe, which makes great use of the beneficial capsaicin.

Homemade Salsa

4 cups chopped fresh tomatoes
1/4 cup chopped green onions
1/2 cup chopped fresh cilantro
3 T pureed garlic
1 T chopped fresh oregano
2 T chopped fresh peppers (as hot as you like it)
1 each red, yellow green pepper, chopped
2 T oil
1/4 cup fresh lemon juice
salt and pepper to taste

Stir all ingredients together in a bowl. Let chill overnight for the flavors to mellow.

Pineapple

Pineapple is a great digestive aid, and the juice has soothing anti-inflammatory properties, thanks to bromelain, an enzyme that helps to digest microbes in the bronchial tubes. It also offers vitamins C, B complex and A. Magnesium, manganese, potassium and copper can also be found alongside pineapple's healthy omega 3 to 6 ratio.

In addition to the nutrients above, pineapple also serves as a healthy source of fiber and enzymes. Since heat can destroy bromelain, a beneficial enzyme, the best way to consume pineapple is raw, as in this fruity salsa, but be sure to eat it fresh for the best enzyme benefits.

Pineapple Mango Salsa

2 cups pineapple chopped
1 cup mango, chopped
4 jalapenos, chopped
1 small onion, finely chopped
1/4 cup chopped cilantro
dash garlic salt

Combine all ingredients in a small bowl. Optional: chill overnight so the flavors can mellow and blend. Serve along with chips as a dip or over grilled chicken.

Pine Nuts

These nuts, which really do come from pine trees, are grown around the world. They are also often called pinon or pignoli nuts or seeds. They are a great source of nutrients, including protein and healthy fats, like most other nuts. Pine nuts also offer vitamins E, K and B complex, iron, magnesium, phosphorus, potassium, zinc copper and manganese. In fact, 1 cup of pine nuts provides nearly 600% of the RDA for manganese! They do have an unhealthy omega 3 to 6 ratio, making them slightly inflammatory. For this reason, a healthy diet should keep pine nuts in moderation. I like this recipe as a classic example on how to include this pricey nut into a meal, as a small flavor contribution, not a main feature.

Orzo with Chicken and Pine Nuts

1 pound tri colored orzo
1/2 cup garlic vinaigrette
1/4 cup chopped sun dried tomatoes
1/4 cup pine nuts
2-3 T shredded Parmesan cheese
2 chicken breasts, cooked and sliced into strips
1 can olives

Cook the pasta and drain off the water. Place into a serving bowl. Add all the remaining ingredients except for the nuts and cheese. Mix well. Top with the cheese then the nuts. Chill overnight to allow the flavors to mellow. Serve cool as a main dish with green salad and crusty bread. (Optional, substitute artichoke hearts for the chicken to make a vegetarian dish.)

Pintos

The pinto bean is a common bean in south-western cooking, especially the American version of Mexican food. Like other beans, the pinto is full of protein, yet fairly low in fat. One cup offers nearly 3/4 of the RDA for folate, making it a great protein source for women of childbearing age. It also offers over half the RDA for fiber and tryptophan, an amino acid that became fairly well know as the soothing, calming turkey ingredient. This amino acid helps to relieve anxiety and is often supplemented in the diets of those that struggle with anxiety or social fears.

Pintos also benefit the body with manganese, protein, phosphorus, iron, magnesium, potassium, copper, and thiamin. Like all beans, pintos offer a healthy amount of fiber, which can help to lower blood pressure. In addition, you can find over 170% of the RDA for molybdenum, a trace mineral that is a key component of the enzyme sulfite oxidase, which is responsible for detoxifying sulfites. Sulfites are often found in cold cuts and processed meats such as hot dogs and can be harmful to the body when not promptly dealt with.

Perhaps the most popular way to consume pintos is in this classic recipe for refried beans. By making them yourself, you can be sure that there are no animal fats or unhealthy oils added to the beans, ensuring maximum health benefits.

Refried Beans

1 cup dried pintos
1T olive oil
1 T garlic puree
1/2 T sea salt
1 t chili powder
1 t onion powder
1 t cumin
1 t lemon juice

Cook the beans with 3 cups of water and a dash of salt in a saucepan. In another pan, add the remaining ingredients and sauté in the oil. Add the beans and 1 cup of the water from the beans. Mash with a fork and cook over low heat about 10 minutes until well combined. Serve with chips and cheese or tortillas and salsa.

Pistachio

This bright green nut is hard to forget, thanks to its distinctive color. These nuts, often called "happy nuts" or "smiling nuts" are native to the Middle Eastern countries and said to be one of the oldest nuts cultivated. In addition to protein and fat, these nuts offer vitamins A, C, E, K, and B complex, calcium, magnesium, copper, phosphorus, iron, potassium, sodium, zinc, and selenium. They are mildly anti-inflammatory, despite having a less than stellar omega 3 to 6 ratio.

Pistachio Chevre Spread

5 ounces of goat cheese
2 T organic butter, softened
1 t garlic puree
1/4 cup pistachios, chopped
salt and pepper to taste

Mix all ingredients together until combined. Serve chilled with vegetable slices, pita wedges or crusty bread slices.

Plantain

Reminiscent of the banana (and often called the cooking banana), the plantain is actually consumed and used in an entirely different way. Native to and most widely used in Latin American cuisine, plantains are not typically consumed raw, unlike bananas. Instead, they are cooked or fried. They offer vitamins A and C, potassium and fiber. They are also slightly astringent and soothing to the digestive tract.

Plantain Syrup

Take 3 plantains and slice into rounds (after peeling). Place into a saucepan with 1/2 cup apple juice, 1/2 cup cranberry juice, 2 T honey and 1 t cinnamon. Bring to a boil, then lower heat to a mild simmer.

Cook until the liquid is reduced into a syrup, about an hour to an hour and a half, stirring 3-4 times an hour. Serve as a dessert sauce over pound cake, angel food cake or even plain ice cream.

Plum

Though my son likes to refer to plums as "the big blueberries," plums are actually similar to a peach or cherry. They grow on every occupied continent, and have a long history as an ancient food. They offer vitamins A, B complex and C, as well as fiber and potassium. While they don't offer a long list of recognized benefits, they do have an impressive array of other beneficial actions.

Plums are rich in phenols, protecting our bodies from free radicals. They also aid digestion and cleanse the liver. Yet, they do contain a high amount of oxalates, which may mean that they can deplete calcium from the body if eaten in large amounts.

Another medicinal use for plums is to dry them out, call them prunes and use them as a laxative, which is a use they are well suited for. Recently, however, prunes got a makeover. It seems the modern generation does not really gravitate towards a food called prunes. So, in the United States, over 10 million dollars were spent transforming the prune to the dried plum. Despite the new image state side, other parts of the world were content with prunes and did not feel any need to change the name. So, the dried plum is an American oddity, while the classic prune still enjoys its popularity elsewhere.

Plums grace many dishes with their rich and bold flavor. I enjoy fish with a dark, deep plum sauce. I also enjoy the lighter side of plums, as in this apple plum butter, which can bring this dinner fruit to the breakfast table.

Plum Butter

Take 2 pounds of pitted and chopped plums, 2 pounds of apples, also chopped, 2 cups of organic apple juice and 2 t cinnamon (optional) and place into a heavy saucepan. Bring to a boil, and boil for 50 to 60 minutes, stirring intermittently. About half way through, check to be sure the fruit is soft and begin to mash it when stirring. After it is all cooked well and the butter is thickened, ladle into prepared canning jars. Seal and store or serve with breakfast breads.

Pomegranate

As it turns out, fruits and vegetables still find their way into fad diets and in and out of popularity. Fortunately for the pomegranate, they are currently on the A-list. They enjoy their 15 minutes of fame, thanks to the large amount of antioxidants they provide. Classically, the pomegranate was a symbol of fertility as an aphrodisiac. The little seeds, while difficult to reach, offer a bright red, tangy juice. Unlike just about any other food, the pomegranate is composed of tart and tangy seeds, which offer their main nutrients.

In addition to their antioxidants, pomegranates help to cleanse the blood, strengthen and soothe the digestive system, and spice up just about any dish. They also offer vitamins C and B complex, iron and potassium. While they can be consumed raw, in fruit salads and as a dessert flavoring, my favorite way to enjoy their deep yet mellow flavor is combined with chicken, like in this recipe. This balsamic glaze is also prefect for holiday turkey dishes; it is one of my favorites.

1 cup pomegranate juice
1/4 cup chopped green onions
2 T olive oil
1/2 cup chicken broth
1/4 cup balsamic vinegar
1 T honey
1 T cornstarch
1 T fresh chopped basil
salt and pepper to taste

Place all ingredients into a saucepan and simmer for 5 minutes until condensed. For added effect, toss in some fresh pomegranate seeds. Serve over freshly grilled chicken or a roasted turkey.

Popcorn

Before popcorn became the movie theater junk food standby, it was a healthy Native American snack. In fact, this snack is still primarily an American obsession. Popcorn is simply corn that has a tough hull and endosperm. When heated, steam collects inside, building up pressure until it literally explodes. Popcorn is high in protein and low in calories, when popped naturally. It is considered a whole grain food and a great source of fiber.

Since the kernels pose a choking hazard, the AAP (American Academy of Pediatrics) does not recommend popcorn as a snack for infants or toddlers. However, the National Cancer Institute and American Diabetes Association both recommend popcorn as a healthy snack for everyone else, primarily due to the healthy fiber content and low glycemic index.

Aside from the classic popped snack with butter and salt, popcorn also is the base of fun snacks known as popcorn balls and candied popcorn. While traditionally unhealthy, this recipe makes a great alternative that will both satisfy your sweet cravings and your commitment to real foods.

Simply take 1 cup unpopped popcorn, pop it, stir in 1.5 cups of pecans and set aside. Meanwhile, take 1 cup of maple syrup and bring to a boil in a saucepan. Cook for about 5 minutes. The foam should thin out and the syrup will darken slightly. Quickly pour over the popcorn and nuts, stirring vigorously. Pour out onto waxed paper and scatter the clumps so they don't stick together. Let cook, then store what hasn't been eaten in an airtight container.

Potatoes

Potatoes are another example of a food we love to hate, mainly due to the common methods of preparation, which include the addition of multiple unhealthy ingredients. Potatoes are one of the world's most popular foods, but this is largely in the form of fried potatoes.

While potatoes can be prepared as a junk food, they can also be prepared as a healthy part of a balanced diet. A medium sized potato served with the skin intact offers roughly 100 calories, plenty of fiber, potassium, chromium, vitamin C and B complex, and even a little protein. The best ways to eat potatoes are baked, broiled and grilled. Since most of our preparations include large amounts of oil or dairy, the best way to make a potato healthier is to go lightly in the addition of fat. My favorite way of adding potatoes to a meal is with this **roasted red potato** recipe.

Take a pound of small red potatoes, scrub them and halve them. Toss in a roasting pan. Drizzle about 2 T olive oil over the top then generously toss in about 1/4 cup fresh herbs. (For the herbs, use what you have on hand, but I always like to include rosemary.) Bake at 400 degrees for about 45 minutes, depending on the size of the potatoes. They should be tender and cooked through, but not falling apart. Serve with sprigs of fresh rosemary.

Poultry

Chicken, turkey, and game hens all fall in this category. Poultry is known as the modern healthy animal protein source for good reason. It is versatile, working with flavors and spices from all regions. It is readily available and affordable. It can be easily prepared as a low fat and high protein dish and has endless cooking options. In addition to protein, you can expect to find niacin, potassium, phosphorus, selenium and zinc from most types of poultry.

As an animal product, poultry still contains cholesterol, animal fat and, depending on the portion of meat, it can be a high fat food. Yet, as far as animal products go, poultry is arguably the best protein source, aside from fish.

Poultry can be grilled, baked, broiled, and roasted, as traditionally served during the winter holidays. It can be chopped into nuggets or fingers, with endless finger food possibilities. My favorite way is over the grill with a little seasoning. This basil Parmesan chicken can be easily made into skewers for a party or left whole for a family dinner.

Basil Parmesan Chicken

Take 4 free range chicken breasts. Sprinkle with salt and pepper and set aside. Mix together 1/4 cup butter, 1/4 cup grated Parmesan cheese, 1 T dried basil and 1 t dried parsley. Bring 2 T of the mixture to the grill with you. As the chicken cooks, brush basil butter over the top. Serve with a scoop of the remaining butter and fresh basil sprigs. The left over butter can be reserved for next time or served with crusty bread.

Pumpkin

When I was a little girl, my daddy used to call my siblings and me his little pumpkins. Each fall, he would head out to the store and return with a bag of orange colored candies in a pumpkin shape with a green top for his little "pumpkins." Those may be the only pumpkins I ate as a child, as I was quite the picky eater, so I avoided most vegetables. However, I later learned that I was not *getting out* of eating them, I was *missing out*.

Pumpkins are great for holiday pies, jack o lanterns, and warming soups. They offer zinc, selenium, vitamins A, C and E, folate, calcium, iron, magnesium and potassium. If you have been paying attention, you also know by now that pumpkins contain loads of healthy antioxidants in the form of that orange pigment beta carotene. This helps to protect against cancers, heart disease and even aging.

Since pumpkin soup and pie recipes abound, I am including a recipe that is great for your little pumpkins that, like me, may need a little convincing when it comes to orange foods!

Pumpkin Spice Cake

1 and a half sticks organic butter, softened
1 and a half cups sucanat
2 cups pumpkin puree (canned is fine, but use organic)
1 t pure vanilla
3 eggs
1 T lemon juice
3 cups wheat flour
1/2 t baking powder
2 t baking soda (aluminum free)
1/2 t salt
1 t cinnamon
1/2 t ground ginger
1/2 t ground cloves
1/2 cup milk

Cream together the butter and sugar. Add the eggs, one at a time. Then add the pumpkin, lemon, milk and vanilla and mix until blended. Add the dry ingredients, 1 cup at a time. Once fully mixed, pour into 3 greased 9 inch pans. Bake at 350 degrees for 20-25 minutes or until golden brown.

For a holiday treat, stack the layers together with this maple cream cheese frosting between each. Mix together one 8 ounce block of cream cheese and 4 t maple syrup. Frost the tops, but not sides, for a rustic stacked look.

Quince

Though historically a highly popular fruit, chances are, you have never seen a quince. They are often called "squashed pears" or the "ugly duckling of the apple family." However ugly their exterior may be, the blossoms produced by this firm fruit are some of the most beautiful of all flower blossoms.

This ancient fruit is slightly astringent, and the high amounts of pectin it contains can help treat diarrhea, if given in small amounts. Quince is low in fat and high in fiber, copper, and vitamin C.

To boost the flavor and nutritional value of a simple sugar syrup, add a little minced quince in during the boiling process. Though, if you are fortunate enough to get your hands on a few, you may prefer to make this classic quince paste, which is traditionally sliced and served with a rich cheese.

Simply take 4 pounds of quinces, peeled and diced. Place in a saucepan with a stick of cinnamon and just enough water to cover the top. Boil for 15 minutes until the fruit is tender. Discard the cinnamon. Blend the quince until smooth and return to the pan with 2-3 cups of sugar. Cook about 20 minutes until it turns a light brown color, then remove and pour into a greased mold to set.

Quinoa

Although not a true cereal grain, quinoa (pronounced keen-wah) has always been revered as an ancient grain. It is a hardy plant as it can tolerate extreme temperatures and thrive in some of the worst conditions. It is easily digested, making it an ideal protein source and easy addition to any diet. It has the highest protein content of any grain, and the WHO (World Health Organization) states that quinoa has as much protein as equal parts of milk. Interestingly enough, its amino acid profile is also similar to milk, which is highly unusual in a plant product. It actually contains more calcium than milk and also offers iron, phosphorus, vitamins B complex and E, manganese and magnesium.

Additionally, quinoa is a great source of lysine, an amino acid that can be difficult to obtain through plant sources. Lysine is essential for tissue growth and repair.

Quinoa is a great food for migraine sufferers. The magnesium content helps to relax the blood vessels, which helps to prevent the constriction characteristic of migraines. Those who suffer from frequent migraines will be happy to hear that increased intake of magnesium has been shown to reduce the frequency of headache episodes. This same mineral also helps with high blood pressure and other cardiovascular diseases, and magnesium deficiencies are not uncommon among those who consume typical modern diets.

Unlike other small sized grain dishes such as couscous or rice, quinoa slightly crunchy after being cooked, adding an interesting texture to the meal. It is also naturally quick cooking, making it an ideal last minute addition. Quinoa can be substituted for rice, couscous or other grains or pastas in most dishes, or try one designed specifically for quinoa, like this Mediterranean quinoa and feta salad.

Quinoa and Feta Salad

1 cup quinoa
1/4 cup chopped fresh Mediterranean herbs (basil, oregano, rosemary…)
3 chopped celery stalks
1 cup halved seedless red grapes
1/4 cup chopped sun dried tomatoes
2/3 cup crumbled feta
3 T vinaigrette (try red wine, citrus or Italian)

Cook quinoa according to package directions. Place into a serving bowl with the herbs, celery, grapes, tomatoes and cheese. Add the vinaigrette and toss to coat. Serve chilled.

Radicchio

This Italian vegetable is also commonly called Italian chicory. The bright red color with white streaks adds variety to a salad of baby greens. It is a blood purifier and digestive aid, increasing bile production. It is low on calories, yet high in magnesium, potassium, calcium and vitamin A. Toss some into your next salad for a spark of color and a crunchy slightly bitter taste.

Radish

This originally obscure vegetable was cultivated in ancient Egypt in the days of the pharaohs. It did not expand its horizons for several centuries, but has now made its way around the globe. Not only do radishes stimulate the appetite, they are a great digestive aid. They provide large amounts of fiber and vitamin C. They also offer a little iron, calcium, potassium, manganese, magnesium, folate and protein.

Radishes are typically used in the Western countries as a digestive aid in a first course salad. They lend themselves nicely to food artists and their carving skills. They also blend nicely with these root vegetables for a savory side dish.

Roasted Root Vegetables

2 cups carrots sliced 1 inch thick
2 cups red potatoes, cubed
1 cup red onions, chopped
3 cups radishes
1 T garlic puree
2 T olive oil
salt and pepper to taste
1 t Mediterranean herb blend

Toss vegetables with oil and spices. Bake in roasting pan at 400 degrees for 45 minutes until vegetables are tender. Serve warm.

Raisin

Prior to the widespread use and importation of cane sugar, raisins were commonly used as sweeteners, second only to honey. This is an effective option because grapes only lose water when they are dehydrated to produce raisins. This concentrates the sweet sugar those fruits are so famous for. They are also easily preserved, a valuable feature of any food.

Since grapes are a heavily sprayed fruit, modern day raisins can also be a concentrated source of pesticides and other toxins. To avoid this, organic raisins are a must-have

Despite the downsides, raisins offer a great nutritional profile. They offer fiber, protein, vitamins C, B complex and K, calcium, iron, magnesium, potassium, manganese, copper, phosphorus and zinc.

Raisins are an easy and tasty addition to many baked goods, but they also hold their own in a trail mix, granola, or even as the main event for an after school snack. I like them best in a breakfast bar like this recipe.

Raisin Oat Bars

1 cup whole wheat flour
1/2 cup rolled oats
1/4 cup sucanat
1/4 cup butter
1/4 cup honey or maple syrup
1 egg
1/2 t pure vanilla
1/2 t baking powder
1/2 t cinnamon
1 cup raisins
optional: 1/2 cup chopped nuts

Mix all ingredients together and press into a square baking pan (greased). Bake at 350 degrees for 20 minutes until lightly browned. Remove, cool and cut into bars. Makes 16 squares or 8 full size bars.

Raspberry

This bright bramble is a favorite of mine. The sweet tart flavor is a highlight of every summer and I eagerly anticipate the berry season every year. Raspberries purify the kidneys and strengthen the liver. They are also great for diarrhea and the leaves are a staple of female preventative care. Red raspberry leaf tea is a uterine tonic that many American midwives use for not only well woman care, but also pregnancy and birth as well.

One cup of fresh raspberries offers nearly 2/3 of the RDA for manganese, half the RDA for vitamin C and a third of your daily fiber. They also offer folate and other B vitamins, magnesium and potassium. They are a rich source of antioxidants, preventing damage to cell membranes and maintaining a healthy internal flora. Raspberries are a great way to keep Candida in check. Raspberries also offer cancer protection and prevent macular degeneration!

To add some of this healthy fruit to the diet, fresh berries can be tossed into a smoothie, onto a batch of pancakes or into any morning baked good. These raspberry almond bars are a great way to add some healthy fats, proteins and a few antioxidants into the diet. They also make an easy breakfast on the go!

Raspberry Almond Bars

1 cup whole wheat flour
1 cup rolled oats
1 cup chopped almonds
1/3 cup almond flour
1 cup organic butter
1 egg

Mix all ingredients together. The dough will resemble coarse crumbs. Divide into half and press one half into an 8 inch square pan that has been thoroughly greased. Bake at 350 degrees for 15 minutes until the crust begins to firm up. Top with a cup of raspberry preserves (the kind that is 100% fruit) and drop the remaining dough in clumps over the top. Bake for an additional 25-30 minutes until the crust is golden brown.

Rhubarb

This unique vegetable is perhaps best known for its relationship with the strawberry. It seems that any rhubarb preparation includes the use of strawberries. This is probably because they not only share a peak harvest season, but their sweet tart combination is a perfect match. The celery-like stalks are 95% water, but rhubarb still offers a nice assortment of nutrients including potassium, vitamins A and C, calcium and fiber.

Rhubarb is also full of tannins, giving it astringent properties. It is good for the liver and functions as a detoxification vegetable. It also contains large amounts of oxalic acid, which can lead to kidney stones and decreased calcium absorption.

Oxalic acid is found naturally occurring in many foods. It is a poisonous colorless substance that many agree is harmless in small quantities, but is harmful in larger amounts. Oxalates are commonly found in berries, grapes, figs, almonds, cashews, peanuts, soy products, quinoa, parsley, chocolate, tea and many other foods. For most individuals, this means nothing.

However, for some, oxalates should be avoided. This is primarily due to the risk of kidney stones and a minor risk of reduced calcium absorption. The problem is that the science just is not clear on the actual harm from these substances. Many respected individuals conclude that there is little to no risk, while others insist there is great risk.

Rice

Rice is the primary staple food for a whopping two thirds of the world. In many countries, the average annual rice consumption is 100 pounds per person. As a complex carbohydrate, rice provides plenty of energy in the diet. It also offers fiber, which aids in healthy digestion, and an assortment of B vitamins.

Rice can also provide iron, protein, calcium, phosphorus and potassium. It is also just as famous for what it does not have, which includes gluten, cholesterol, sodium and fat.

Rice has a natural hull surrounding it for protection, but this hull is inedible, so it must be removed. The differences in how rice is processed from this point are outlined in this excerpt from the *World's Healthiest Foods* website:

> "The process that produces brown rice removes only the outermost layer, the hull, of the rice kernel and is the least damaging to its nutritional value. The complete milling and polishing that converts brown rice into white rice destroys 67% of the vitamin B3, 80% of the vitamin B1, 90% of the vitamin B6, half of the manganese, half of the phosphorus, 60% of the iron, and all of the dietary fiber and essential fatty acids. Fully milled and polished white rice is required to be "enriched" with vitamins B1, B3 and iron."

Obviously, brown rice is the best source of nutrients. White rice, like other refined foods, should not be considered to be an acceptable alternative. There are plenty of alternatives for whole rice that can be adjusted to suit any dish. Many add color, flavor and texture such as basmati, arborio, black, pecan, red, and others. The only exception is wild rice, which is not actually a rice and will be covered later in this section.

Different types of rice can easily be added to just about any entrée. Rice is typically served with beans, which complement its amino acid profile. Rice and beans combine to create a complete protein. Since rice is such a versatile food, I've provided examples of two completely different ways to serve it. First up is a traditional Italian vegetarian dish, arancini. Then, with the leftover rice, you can make a classic side dish or light meal, fried rice.

Arancini

1/2 cup Panko bread crumbs
8-10 small fresh mozzarella balls
4 cups brown rice
1 t pureed garlic
3 T cup onions, finely chopped
1 egg
1/2 cup Parmesan cheese
1 cup marinara sauce

Cook the rice in a rice cooker or stovetop with the garlic and onions according to package directions. Divide rice in half and set half aside. This will be saved for the fried rice recipe later. Take the other half and mix in the Parmesan cheese and egg. Take each mozzarella ball and cover completely with the rice mixture. Be sure to completely encase the cheese. Roll the large balls in the bread crumbs and place on a baking sheet. Bake at 400 degrees for 20-25 minutes, until the bread crumbs are crisp and browned. Spoon the marinara sauce onto 4 dinner plates and place the arancini over the bed of sauce. Serve warm with crusty bread and a green salad.

Fried Rice

2 eggs
2 cups leftover brown rice (cooked)
1 cup vegetables (chopped carrots, celery, green peas etc.)
salt and pepper to taste
3 T tamari (soy sauce)

Crack the eggs in a medium pan over medium heat. Stir them as scrambled eggs. When they begin to cook, add the rice and stir well. Cook about 5 minutes until rice is warmed thoroughly. Add the vegetables and cook until tender. Stir in the seasonings and serve warm.

Romaine

Romaine is arguably the most popular dinner salad green, gracing dinner buffets and family tables nightly. It can be found with both green and red leaves and makes a hearty base for any salad topping. It is crisp, yet full of nutrients such as iron and fiber. Romaine offers over 150% of the RDA for vitamin K. It also provides vitamin A, chromium, potassium, B complex, calcium and protein.

Like all lettuces, romaine regularly holds a space on the "dirty dozen", a list put out by the EWG (Environmental Working Group) of the 12 foods that have been found to be most contaminated by pesticides. These residues are difficult to remove, making organic the best buy for any lettuce.

Maple Bleu Cheese Salad

2 cups red romaine leaves
2 cups green romaine leaves
1/2 cup sliced red onion
1 green apple, chopped
2 stalks celery, chopped
1/2 cup crumbled bleu cheese
1/2 cup pecans
2 T maple syrup

In a small saucepan over medium heat, toss the pecans with the maple syrup. Cook until the syrup is absorbed and crystallizes around the pecans. Set aside to cool. Meanwhile, make the **Dijon vinaigrette** with:

1/4 cup maple syrup
1/4 cup apple cider vinegar
1/3 cup extra virgin olive oil
1 t stone ground mustard
dash salt and pepper

Whisk all ingredients together and set aside. Place the greens onto a large serving plate and top with all the salad toppings, finishing with the bleu cheese. Drizzle 1/4 cup vinaigrette over the top before serving and save the rest of the dressing for later.

Rutabaga

While rutabagas are often considered to be yellow turnips, they are, in reality, a cross between wild cabbage and turnips. These cruciferous vegetables offer a multitude of nutrients, including calcium, copper, iron, magnesium, manganese, phosphorus, potassium and selenium. They also offer vitamins A, B complex, C, and E. Like other root vegetables, they cleanse the liver, aid in digestion and strengthen the stomach.

Like turnips, rutabagas can be added to soups, stews, stir fry or steamed meats. They can also be consumed raw, in a slaw dish and in carrot salad. I like them with an assortment of colors in a **roasted root vegetable** dish, which adds not only color, but also valuable nutrients to any holiday table.

2 cups red onions
4 cups baby red potatoes, halved
1 cup rutabagas, cut into cubes
1 cup carrots, cut into 1 inch slices
2 T butter
dash salt and pepper
1 T dried Mediterranean herbs
1 t pureed garlic

Toss all ingredients into a large roasting pan. Be sure butter and herbs are well blended into the vegetables. Bake at 400 degrees for 45-60 minutes until vegetables are tender.

Rye

Rye is one of the newest grains. This slightly tangy grain comes from a robust plant that can hold up quite well, even in harsh conditions. Rye offers a nutritional profile similar to wheat, but with less gluten. It also offers quite a bit of the amino acid lysine, which can be difficult to obtain from plant sources. You can also find B vitamins, iron, protein, and other nutrients in rye.

While commonly used for whiskey making, rye is most popular for the tangy bread and filling sandwiches that it can produce. It lends itself well to naturally leavened breads, as rye ferments quite easily. Try it out in this recipe.

Natural Rye Bread

2 cups rye flour
1 and 1/2 cup bread flour
1 T caraway seeds
1 cup sourdough bread starter
1 T olive oil
1/2 t sea salt
1 T molasses

Feed the starter with 1 cup of the rye and 1/2 cup water. Leave for 12 hours in a warm spot. Add the remaining ingredients and knead to form a smooth dough. Place in a medium bowl, cover and let rise 4-6 hours or until doubled. Punch down, shape into 2 loaves and place into 2 greased loaf pans. Let rise again, 2-3 hours or until a nice round shape has formed. Bake at 350 degrees for 20 minutes. Open the oven, brush with water, then bake an additional 25 minutes or until golden.

Safflower Oil

This polyunsaturated vegetable oil is closely related to sunflower oil. It is inexpensive when compared to other oils. It is also extremely heat stable, and anti-inflammatory. With all these qualifications, safflower oil generally gets a reputation as a heart healthy oil. Nonetheless, it contains all omega 6 fatty acids, with no omega 3s. While most cooking and table oils contain more omega 6 fatty acids than omega 3s, this complete lack is certainly a drawback. In addition to the 14 fat grams per tablespoon, the oil contains vitamins E and K.

Safflower oil can still be included in the healthy diet, as long as these caveats are taken into consideration. If the oil comes from plants that have not been genetically modified, the heat stability comes in handy in the modern kitchen, especially when trying to avoid the toxins that come from rancid oils.

Sea Salt

Since most common table salt comes from deep within the earth, the soft, subtler flavor of sea salt is often preferred among gourmet chefs. Plain sea salt contains a mineral content similar to that of plain mined salt. Mineral sea salt, however still retains the minerals that are found along with the salt in the sea and is a healthier option than plain salts. These minerals are also more bioavailable than many mineral supplements.

Sodium is an essential mineral, yet is commonly found in overabundance in many diets. It is one of the important electrolytes and is essential to health. It is also found in unbalanced ratios (with potassium) in processed foods. Contrary to popular belief, there is a difference between plain table salt and organic sodium. The intense heat with which table salt is processed causes the sodium molecules to split, greatly reducing the bioavailability of the sodium. This sodium, however, closely resembles the sodium our body needs, which can trick the body into storing it for use. This excess stored sodium can contribute to health problems such as high blood pressure. Natural, bioavailable sodium, however, can assist with calcium availability and the pH of the body. Only high quality sea salts qualify as a whole food for health purposes. Other sea salts and plain table salt should be only in the diet in very limited quantities.

Seaweed

Seaweed may come as a bit of a surprise under the heading of whole foods, since many of us have childhood memories of seaweed as nothing more than a nuisance during our beach vacations. Nonetheless, this sea vegetable, as it is often called, can be a valid part of a healthy diet. Like sea water, sea vegetables are a rich source of minerals. In addition to the strengthening properties found in the minerals, seaweed helps to reduce cholesterol, detoxify the body and even offers antibiotic properties. It also plays a vital role in the production of many high quality beauty products.

As one of the richest source of nutrients in the diet, seaweed offers calcium, iodine, phosphorus, sodium, iron, protein, and vitamins A, B complex, C and E. The iodine content is beneficial for thyroid issues, specifically hypothyroidism, which can be caused by a lack of iodine.

While a common concern about seaweed lies in the pollution content of our oceans, many laboratory tests have shown this pollution is not concentrated in seaweed. Though the evidence is hardly conclusive, it appears seaweed is free from these contaminants. Seaweed can easily be incorporated into the diet, especially if the diet is already rich in Japanese or similar foods.

In addition to its usefulness in soups and as a sushi wrap, seaweed can be purchased crushed in a shaker as a condiment. When consumed in this way, it is easily added to just about any recipe. To try this easy method, place a shaker of seaweed near the stove. Keep it in mind, and you will find plenty of dishes that can be improved with this nutrient rich food.

Seitan

This vegetarian meat alternative is pronounced SAY-tahn. Seitan is actually wheat gluten, which, if you recall, is a rich protein source. It is a common meat substitute among vegetarians, especially in China, Russia and Southeast Asia. Like tofu, seitan is fairly flavorless and can take on the flavor of the spices and herbs that are used in the dish. While gluten is certainly a rich source of protein, I strongly hesitate to recommend it as a protein source due to the increasing intolerances to gluten. One in 133 individuals have celiac disease, which is the name for a lifelong gluten intolerance, but many experts believe the actual number is quite a bit higher as the disorder is extremely undiagnosed and the available testing is often inaccurate. Considering this, I feel there are plenty of better options for vegetarian protein sources.

Sesame

These tiny seeds are reported to be one of the oldest foods known to man. Useful for their oil as well as nutritional value, they find themselves in far more foods than most realize. These seeds can be found sprinkled over the tops of many baked goods, and the ground seeds or butter, called tahini, are an important ingredient in hummus.

While sesame seeds are a great source of calcium, this calcium is tightly bound to oxalic acid, making it unavailable. They do, however, offer plenty of protein, oil, iron, phosphorus and B complex vitamins. Due to the many chemicals that are typically used to process sesame seeds, only organic seeds should be added to the healthy diet.

Shallots

Shallots are close relatives to both garlic and onions. Garlic and onions are both known for adding a strong odor and taste to a dish, while shallots provide a milder, somewhat sweeter flavor. They are perfect for recipes that call for onions, but need a mild flavor. Shallots still provide many of the great health benefits found in garlic and onions, but without the powerful punch of flavor. I like to use them in sauces for grilled or roasted meats.

Versatile Shallot Reduction

1 shallot, diced
1/2 cup red or white wine (white for poultry and fish; red for other meats - if avoiding wine, any type of stock can be used instead)
2 T butter
1 T olive oil
salt and pepper to taste

Place a saucepan over medium heat and warm the olive oil. Add the shallot and sauté until tender, but not brown - about 3-4 minutes. Add the wine or stock and reduce heat to a simmer. Continue to simmer until the liquid is reduced by half. Add the butter, salt and pepper and whisk until glossy and smooth. Pour over freshly grilled meat and serve immediately.

Sorghum

Growing up in Alabama, the only time I heard the word sorghum as a child was when it was quickly followed by the word molasses. I basically assumed sorghum was a type of sugarcane until I began to study nutrition. Sorghum is actually an ancient grain, similar to millet. It has a mild, sweet flavor and is gluten free. As a grain, it offers plenty of B vitamins, iron, protein and calcium. You may find it under the marketing name "jowar" in the grocery store.

Now, on to the best part: the molasses. More than likely, sorghum molasses is the most readily available food product you will find from this plant. Sorghum molasses was the sweetener of choice a couple of hundred years ago when refined sugar was much less common. It is unfortunate that it does not retain that place in our homes today. Sorghum molasses is made from the sorghum stalk and has a taste similar to regular molasses, but a nutrient content much like that of blackstrap molasses. You can expect plenty of iron, B vitamins and calcium from sorghum molasses. There are plenty of great ways to add sorghum molasses to the diet. The classic way is to pour it over freshly baked buttermilk biscuits. It can also be used anywhere you would another liquid sweetener. Try pancakes, waffles, French toast, etc. The possibilities are endless.

Soybeans

Soybeans are a tricky topic to cover in this small space. They are a health food. Yet, they can be harmful. The most important thing to remember when studying soy is balance. The soybean is a little Asian pea packed with protein. It contains isoflavones, which are plant estrogens that have been credited with stalling osteoporosis, alleviating menstrual problems and preventing cancer. While it offers an impressive laundry list of qualifications, there are also downsides to this little plant.

One major concern is that soy is one of the most genetically engineered foods today. It is imperative to only purchase certified organic soy products to ensure your soy is not a chemical concoction of modifications and indirect additives. Another concern is that soy inhibits certain valuable enzymes when prepared the typical western way.

Without diving head first into a lengthy debate on the pros and cons of soy, the bottom line is that soy can be a healthy addition to the diet. Fermented soy products, such as tempeh and soy sauce, are the healthiest ways to consume the food, as the enzyme inhibition process is halted. It is also important to remember to keep moderation in mind. Organic fermented soy can be a valuable contribution to the diet, but it should not serve as the focal point of every meal. This is especially common among vegetarians. A proper vegetarian diet is a healthy alternative, but it involves consuming a variety of vegetables, not meat substitutes at every meal. Therefore, while soy adds health benefits to the diet, it is important to ensure that it is consumed only as a part of a balanced diet, not the focal point.

Spinach

Certain sailors will tell you this leafy green vegetable is the ideal food for body builders, but I am more impressed by the cleansing and restorative effects of the plant. As a mild laxative, spinach is an ideal food for maintaining colon health. You can also expect to find plenty of vitamins C, A, E, K and B complex, manganese, potassium, magnesium, iron and even a little bit of protein in the average serving.

While most leafy greens are best served in a salad, spinach is also tasty and nutritious cooked into numerous meals. In springtime, I enjoy a light spinach and strawberry salad, but in the fall and winter, I always prefer a warm, hearty **spanakopita**, which is a nutritious and filling Greek pastry.

2 pounds spinach
1 cup feta cheese
1 T parsley
1 egg
1 stick unsalted butter, melted
salt and pepper to taste
1 pound filo pastry

Thaw the filo sheets, if needed. In a medium bowl, mix together the spinach, feta, egg, parsley, salt and pepper. Unwrap the filo dough and cut into 3 inch strips. Brush with melted butter. Spoon a teaspoon of the spinach mixture into the corner of the strip and begin to fold into a triangle. Continue folding until the entire strip has been used. Brush tops with melted butter. Repeat with remaining strips. Bake for 25 minutes at 350 degrees.

Spirulina

Spirulina, named for its spiral shape, is one of the most primitive food products humans consume. This blue green algae is packed with protein, vitamins A, B complex, and E, iron, and beneficial bacteria (probiotics). Additionally, spirulina is a great source of healthy fats, including the elusive GLA.

In addition to the nutritional benefits, spirulina boosts the immune system, lowers cholesterol and helps to prevent cancer.

Spirulina can be consumed as a supplement, but is best taken as a powder that serves as a condiment. It blends well with water and juice, but also flavors pasta and various energy bars. The Granola Chic, one of my favorite whole foods chefs, serves her kids their own green eggs with spirulina colored eggs flavored with maple syrup.

Sprouts

Sprouts are not a food by themselves, rather a way to consume various beans, grains and legumes. Sprouting foods is a great way to increase the nutritional content. By sprouting seeds, the nutrients are more readily absorbed, and can easily be consumed in just about any dish. Sprouted seeds are also easier to digest, making them a great choice for those with hindered digestive tracts.

The nutrient content varies according to the specific food that has been sprouted. Most sprouts are beneficial in assisting the liver in the detoxification process. They are also rich in fiber, protein, and B complex vitamins. Additionally, sprouts offer plenty of beneficial enzymes for digestion.

Commonly sprouted foods include broccoli seeds, alfalfa, chickpea, lentil, soybean, mung bean and clover. While sprouts can be purchased in health food stores, many families prefer to simply grow their own. This is pretty simple to do with a canning jar, cheesecloth and seeds. Simply soak the seeds in water, then place in the jar with the cloth on top. Allow the seeds to begin to sprout and harvest them.

The tricky thing about sprouts, however, is the potential danger of consuming raw sprouts. While the enzymes are beneficial, both homegrown and store bought sprouts can also harbor harmful bacteria. For this reason, most professionals encourage home sprouters to fully cook their sprouts prior to consumption. While many argue that this kills off many of the beneficial nutrients, and it does, the process should at least be a consideration for pregnant women, those with a weakened immune system, including the elderly, children, and those with both chronic and acute illness.

Squash

When my siblings and I complained about our dinnertime fare as children, my father always reminded me to be grateful I wasn't having squash casserole. Having no idea what such a food could taste like, I knew it had to be terrible if it could serve as a worst case scenario! Imagine my surprise to learn that squash was actually a decent food, and when prepared correctly, a squash casserole has potential to be a tasty dish!

Squash comes in many varieties and is often categorized as summer squash or winter squash, based on seasonal availability. Winter squash include acorn squash, butternut squash and spaghetti squash, while zucchini is an example of a summer squash. They are members of the gourd family, and while the exact nutrient content varies according to the variety, squash in general offers plenty of vitamins A and C. They also contain potassium, fiber, manganese, B complex, and copper. They are rich in phytonutrients, and beneficial in treating enlarged prostates.

Butternut Squash Risotto

1 cup Arborio rice
3 cups vegetable broth
2 cups water
1/2 t onion powder
1/2 t garlic powder
2 T parsley flakes
1/2 t pepper
2 T olive oil
1 small butternut squash (about 1 pound)

Halve the squash and bake at 400 degrees for 25 minutes until tender. Let cool.

Meanwhile, heat the oil over medium heat with the onion, garlic and pepper. Add the rice and stir as it cooks about 2-3 minutes. Add the broth and water, 1/2 cup at a time.

Let the rice almost completely absorb the liquid before adding another 1/2 cup. Total cook time should take about 25 minutes.

Scoop out the inside of the squash and mash with a fork until it is smooth. Add 1/2 cup to finished risotto, along with the parsley. Serve topped with another 1/4 cup squash for garnish.

Starfruit

This fun yellow fruit is an oval citrus fruit that happens to slice into perfectly shaped stars, hence the name. The fruit offers vitamin C and potassium. It also helps to relieve diarrhea.

Star fruit is best consumed raw, and can be eaten with minimal preparation. My favorite use, however, is as a pretty salad garnish. Slice the fruit into individual stars and top a bright green salad with them. Add a tangy vinaigrette and not only do you have a perfect presentation, but the combined nutrient content is highly desirable.

Strawberry

Freshly picked organic strawberries are absolutely unbeatable, and no conventional or processed food can even begin to compete. These flavorful red berries pack a nutritious punch, but their strong bold taste is what often wins the hearts (taste buds?) of children and adults alike. Not only are they rich in antioxidants and mildly detoxifying, strawberries offer vitamin C and B complex, magnesium, and fiber. Their ORAC value is 3520.

Strawberries also have a sedative effect on many, so the aroma is often used in holistic children's dental offices. They help to increase the appetite, and even have some antiviral properties.

Strawberries are best consumed directly off the vine, freshly plucked. If you have never experienced the luxury of consuming fresh organic berries, you must go out and find a local farm next spring! These berries taste like an entirely different food when compared to the bland dull fruits found in grocery stores.

When the berries are ripe, the uses are endless. Medicinally, they can be used to brighten teeth. Have you ever wondered about those harsh chemical tooth whiteners? Strawberries can provide a great alternative. Simply take 3-4 fresh berries and remove the stems. Crush them and mix with 2 T baking soda. Gently brush the mixture onto your teeth, fully coating each tooth. Allow to sit for 4-5 minutes then finish brushing the paste off. This will remove stains from coffee, soda and other food products, but the acid can damage teeth if used more than once or twice a week.

Since these fruits are too delicious to simply apply to our teeth, I've also included a yummy strawberry recipe. Strawberries blend effortlessly into just about any dish. Toss them onto a spinach salad, coat with chocolate for a flawless dessert, or place onto a biscuit with freshly whipped cream. For a quick and easy strawberry topping that is well suited for pancakes, waffles, biscuits or whatever you have on hand, try this recipe.

Strawberry Syrup

2 cups strawberry halves
3 T maple syrup
1/2 t cinnamon
2 T lemon juice
1 t vanilla extract

Mix well and store in a sealed jar in the fridge. Let rest overnight for the flavors to mellow.

Sunflower (seeds and oil)

Sunflowers are some of my favorite flowers. The girly side of me loves that they grow wild, free and tall with beautiful petals and color. The practical side of me can't resist the functional beauty of a sunflower, making sunflowers a must-have in any garden. Fortunately, not only are they easy to grow and beautiful to behold; sunflowers are a highly nutritious food that can and should be a part of a healthy diet.

The seeds offer hefty amounts of protein, even more than beef. They offer fat, but it is the healthy heart promoting kind of fat, which I like to see. You can also find B complex vitamins, manganese, iron, calcium, magnesium, copper, and the amino acid tryptophan in a handful of seeds.

While my daughter loves to eat them by the handful, they can be easily incorporated into any recipe for the skeptic. Simply substitute the seeds for nuts in just about anything from cookies to muffins or even vegetable dishes to introduce the nutty flavor of sunflower seeds to the palate.

As a healthy fat source, sunflowers are also used for their oil content. The oil extracted from the plant has a light nutty taste and is a good source of omega 3 fatty acids. Like other healthy unsaturated oils, it has a short shelf life and becomes oxidized quickly, so it should only be purchased in small amounts, consumed fresh, and never heated.

Crunchy Sunflower Pilaf

1/2 cup sunflower seeds
dash salt
2 T butter
1 cup chicken broth
1/2 cup barley
2/3 cup brown rice

In a rice cooker, place rice and barley with broth and 2.5 cups of water. (Or, cook according to package directions) Remove, fluff with a fork and add seeds, salt, and butter. Top with a dash of black pepper and parsley.

Sweet Potatoes

While technically neither a potato nor a yam, sweet potatoes are often lumped together with both. What they are is sweet, healthy, and delicious. They are native to Central America and are one of the oldest foods known to man.

Sweet potatoes offer antioxidant rich carotenoids (hence the color), vitamins A, C, B complex, copper, potassium, iron and fiber. Despite the association with sugar, sweet potatoes actually help to balance blood sugar levels. In trials, not only did they stabilize blood sugar levels, they also helped to reduce insulin resistance. Additionally, the rich antioxidant content is beneficial for a number of disorders.

Traditionally associated with Thanksgiving, sweet potatoes offer an impressive array of nutrients that are worth giving the vegetable a second look. Try adding them to the diet in this recipe for roasted root vegetables.

Roasted Potato Medley

1 pound each: sweet and white potatoes
Spice blend: 1 t each parsley, garlic salt, onion salt, thyme, rosemary, basil
3 t olive oil

Chop the vegetables into 1-2 inch chunks. Place into a baking pan and drizzle the olive oil over the top. Top with herbs and stir to combine. Place into a preheated 400-degree oven and bake for an hour until the vegetables are cooked and golden brown.

Tangerines

This small mandarin fruit is named after the small Moroccan port where it received its first boost to fame. The dark red fruit is in season during December, so they make a great addition to a Christmas stocking. Their nutrient content does not vary much from other citrus fruits, and can be found under the mandarin heading.

Roasted Chicken with Tangerine Glaze

1 whole chicken
1 of each: onion, carrot, and celery stalk
2 cups chicken stock
3 tangerines
2 t sage
1 t parsley
1 T honey
1 T cornstarch
Salt and pepper to taste

Chop the onion, celery and carrot, then place in a roasting pan. Add the chicken and roast in the oven at 400 degrees, basting every 20 minutes until chicken is not quite done. In a saucepan, combine the juice, honey, herbs, and cornstarch. Bring to a boil and cook until thick, about 2 minutes. Pour over the chicken and place back into the oven until the glaze is browned and glossy. Serve with a rice pilaf.

Tapioca

This flavorless starch comes from the cassava root. It is most known for the pudding it produces, but can also be useful as a glaze or thickener. Like agar, it makes a great substitute for gelatin, especially for vegetarians.

While it has little to offer as far as recognized nutrient content, it is soothing to the digestive tract, making it a perfect healing food for a sore throat or anyone with digestive problems. Since it serves as a base for foods, the added nutrients can vary according to the ingredients. I like it with antioxidant rich pomegranate juice in this bright recipe:

Honeyed Pomegranate Tapioca

1/2 cup tapioca pearls (pre soaked)
2 cups pomegranate juice
2 T honey
1/2 cup milk

Place the pearls into the juice and let soak for an hour. Add the honey and milk, then place over medium heat until it simmers. Allow to simmer for 10-15 minutes until the pearls are soft and thoroughly cooked. Chill overnight. Top with whipped cream.

Tea

Tea is second only to water as the world's most popular beverage, and with good reason. Research shows that both black and green teas have cancer fighting antioxidants, inhibit tumor cell growth, prevent heart disease and strengthen the immune system. Of the two, green tea is the healthier option, as it contains more polyphenols, which are the compounds responsible for much of the medicinal action.

Classic tea comes in many "colors." Black tea, the most common variety, is fermented. The enzymes darken the leaves and the resulting tea has a strong flavor. Green tea has been steamed to deactivate certain enzymes, and then dried. The tea is much more mild in both color and taste. Red tea, also called yellow or oolong, is fermented, but not like black tea. It gives a robust flavor that is stronger than green but not as strong as black. Finally, white tea has only been dried. It has not been steamed or fermented, and the resulting tea is the mildest of all.

All varieties of tea can be flavored with other herbs and flowers to add to the complexity of the flavor. Other additives, such as honey or milk, are also common, but each adds its own nutritional benefits and detriments.

While most individuals benefit from the consumption of tea on a regular basis, some individuals should not regularly consume tea. These individuals are children, those prone to oxalate stones, and those with iron deficiencies.

Tea can be used as a base for just about any drink. Green is my personal favorite, as it is easy to find and offers healthy benefits. It also offers a mellow flavor that can be adjusted to suit just about any palate.

Try experimenting with fruits and juices to create your own masterpiece, or grab one of the recipes below.

Apple Peach Tea
4 cups brewed green tea
2 cups apple juice
2 whole peaches, peeled and diced

Place all ingredients into a blender. Pulse until thoroughly mixed. Feel free to leave as chunky or smooth as you like. Serve cold.

Lemonade Tea
4 cups green tea
Juice of 2 whole lemons
2-3 T sugar

Place all ingredients together in a pitcher and mix well. Be sure sugar is dissolved and serve over ice.

Blackberry Tea
4 cups green tea
1 cup fresh berries
2 T sugar

Mash and strain berries. Stir into the tea along with the sugar (if desired). Be sure ingredients are well mixed and chill overnight to allow the flavors to mellow and deepen. Serve with fresh berries.

Tempeh

Tempeh is a traditional food made by splitting, fermenting and cooking soybeans. It can easily be found in many natural food stores, but is just as easy to make at home. Homemade tempeh is healthier because it contains many nutrients that are not found in the commercial production method. As a rich protein source, it forms the base of many vegetarian entrees.

I find tempeh to be a healthy meal option to include in a varied diet. Unfortunately, some individuals become vegetarians or vegans for health reasons, but instead of changing the diet, they simply substitute soy for meat. They eat the exact same menu with soymilk, soy cheese, tofu, tempeh, and so on. This practice does avoid animal fat and potential health concerns, but replaces it with other potential health detriments. Instead of focusing the diet on a major protein source, these vegetarians would do well to actually consume a varied diet of plant-based nutrients. Too much soy can lead to plenty of health concerns just as quickly as too much meat can.

Having said that, I do find that fermented soy can make a healthy addition to the diet, offering plenty of protein, B vitamins, and omega 3s. It is not consumed raw and can be cooked in just about any manner. It also absorbs spices well and can be transformed into just about any regional dish.

Tofu

Tofu, like tempeh, is a soy protein source that can be used as a meat substitute in vegetarian dishes. Tofu is perhaps the most popular alternative protein source today. Tofu is low in calories, high in protein, and cholesterol free. It is made from curdled soymilk. It can be purchased in a block, which can be sliced or chopped to use in an array of dishes. It can also be easily made at home. Much of the nutritional information is the same as with tempeh, though the two soy foods vary greatly in flavor, texture and preparation. Tempeh is preferable to tofu among many health professionals, as the fermentation process inhibits certain chemical reactions that otherwise naturally occur.

Tomatillo

Commonly mistaken for green tomatoes, tomatillos are actually a different plant entirely, although they are technically in the same family. The little fruits are green and come encased in a paper shell. They offer a tangy flavor to many Mexican meals through the popular green sauce. If a recipe calls for tomatillos and you cannot find them locally, green tomatoes and some lemon juice make an acceptable substitute.

Tomatillos are a low calorie food, offering very little fat, some fiber, magnesium, manganese, copper, niacin, iron and vitamin C. In addition to their unique flavor, their nutrient content makes them a desirable addition to the healthy diet.

Green Salsa

8-10 tomatillos, peeled
4 jalapenos (for mild salsa, remove the seeds)
1 T cilantro
2 t pureed garlic

Place all ingredients in a blender with salt to taste. Chop until thoroughly mixed. Add up to 1/3 cup water, if needed.

Turnips

Turnips grow well in poor soil and under harsh conditions, which has given them a lowly reputation. However, this Eurasia native is not only a beneficial digestive aid, it also is rich in key nutrients. Turnips offer calcium, potassium, vitamins C and B complex, and phosphorus. They also help to detoxify the body.

The key to tasty turnips is to ensure they are ripe, but not overripe. The flavor tends to absorb other flavors, so seasoning is everything when cooking turnips. Care should also be taken not to overcook them. When overcooked, they release a mustard smell that it less than appetizing.

Vanilla

This orchid is probably one of the most exotic foods many individuals consume. It is the only orchid humans consume, and the pollination process actually occurs by hand. Since the pollination has to occur within hours of the flower opening, it is pretty easy to see why vanilla is the second most expensive spice in the world. (Saffron is the most expensive.)

Vanilla is a digestive aid, but the real values lie in the aromatherapy benefits. It is used to boost self-confidence, mellow tempers and relieve frustration.

When buying vanilla, it is key to ensure the extract is a pure extract, not synthetic flavoring. The quality of vanilla extracts varies greatly, which is why the best way to ensure you are using good vanilla is to infuse your own. Make sure to use organic beans. The longer the extract is left to infuse, the more developed the flavor will be.

Vanilla Extract

7 vanilla beans
pint size canning jar
pint of vodka or brandy

Split the beans lengthwise and place in the jar. Pour the alcohol over the top and cap tightly. Store in a dark cabinet for 6-8 weeks. To use: remove the beans and use as vanilla extract in any recipe. Or, leave the beans in the jar to make "perpetual vanilla." After using, refill the jar with additional alcohol. Continually refilling will provide more vanilla extract, with the strength weakening over time.

Vinegar

Vinegar has always been an important food, medicinal agent, preservative, beauty product, etc. The uses of this substance range from cleaning products to exotic gourmet meals. Technically, the word means "sour wine" but vinegar can be made from just about anything that will ferment, including grapes, malt, rice and even apples.

Vinegar is a digestive aid, helps to detoxify the body and strengthen the liver, and can even help with depression. However, not all vinegar is the beneficial kind. Traditionally, vinegar is made by fermenting the foods mentioned above. Modern vinegar, however, is not a whole food. It is often bottled and shipped in mere days. Look for "traditionally fermented vinegar" or "unfiltered" or even "aged in wood." Vinegar should always be stored in glass and cooked in non-reactive metals.

One final note; distilled vinegar is not only on the "non-healthy" list, it actually leaches minerals from the body. It also is likely made from synthetic materials, and should never be consumed, thought it is beneficial when used in homemade cleaning products.

When you do get your hands on wholesome vinegar, it is a great addition to salad dressings and plenty of other recipes. Try it plain or flavored, as in this holiday recipe.

Cranberry Orange Vinegar

1 quart vinegar
2 cups cranberries
1/4 cup honey or maple syrup
1/3 cup orange juice
1T orange zest

Combine all ingredients in a saucepan. Bring to a boil and simmer for 3-5 minutes while berries burst. Remove from heat and chill 3-4 days. Strain the mixture (a wire mesh strainer lined with cheesecloth is ideal) and store in tightly closed jars.

Walnuts

English walnuts (also called Persian walnuts) are the most common nuts in the world. Not to be confused with the American black walnut, these nuts offer anti-inflammatory properties and healthy omega 3 fatty acids. In fact, 1/4 cup of walnuts offers nearly 100% of the RDA for omega 3s. Walnuts also offer manganese, copper and tryptophan.

Other health benefits from walnuts include alleviating hypertension, improving cholesterol ratios, and preventing gallstones. Walnuts also have plenty of naturally occurring melatonin and antioxidants, making them beneficial for all forms of depression and sleep problems. Additionally, despite their high fat content, eating walnuts actually contributes to weight loss. That is probably due to the type of fats naturally occurring in the nuts.

Many of these benefits are diminished in conventional walnuts, which are often bleached, polished, fumigated and treated with gas to produce uniform tan nuts. Look for organic nuts, which will vary in color and size, for best nutritional content.

The best way to eat these walnuts is raw, although they can be baked into just about any bakery treat to boost flavor.

Watermelon

Watermelon, named after its primary ingredient, is the quintessential summer afternoon treat. Native to Africa, this vegetable is over 90% water. Watermelon also has roughly half the sugar an apple has, yet tastes sweeter, making it ideal for dieters.

In addition to its thirst quenching properties, watermelons have plenty to offer in terms of health benefits. First, they are rich in vitamins C, A and B complex, potassium and magnesium. They are packed with antioxidants, protect against macular degeneration, prevent erectile dysfunction, lower blood pressure and increase insulin sensitivity.

These bright melons are best consumed fresh and raw. Watermelon juice is also a tasty way to consume the health benefits. Simply remove the seeds and blend in a blender for a few seconds. The juice is thick, but can be watered down or blended with another juice (such as apple or white grape) for a sweeter drink that resembles what we often think of as "juice".

Wheat / Wheat Grass

Wheat is an ancient grain that forms the base of nearly all modern day breads. Like rice, it is a key source of nutrients, as an estimated 1/3 of the world's population depends on wheat for nourishment. Whole wheat (note the word "whole") offers B complex vitamins, protein, manganese, fiber, tryptophan and vitamin E.

Wheat is generally available in a couple of forms, although there are literally thousands of potential varieties. Hard wheat has a higher gluten content, making it ideal for breads. Soft wheat is lower in gluten, making it more suitable for pastries and cakes. Wheat is also named for the season in which it was sown. Spring wheat is sown in the spring and harvested in the fall, offering a higher gluten content. Winter wheat is generally sown in the fall, germinates, and then grows in the spring. This process usually makes winter wheat richer in minerals.

Whole grains lower the risk of many health problems, including diabetes, gallstones, constipation, colon and breast cancer, childhood asthma, heart disease and weight problems. Many of these benefits are due to the high fiber content, and many of the benefits are even more impressive when the wheat is used in a sourdough preparation. For more details on that, flip back to the Seven Confusing Foods chapter.

Whole grains are often difficult to introduce into a diet that is used to bleached white flour. My favorite way of sneaking them in is to offer them first in a fun treat such as cookies or cakes. This flavorful berry cake is a yummy summer treat and yet still fairly healthy.

Summer Berry Pound Cake with Citrus Glaze

1.5-2 cups white wheat flour
1 cup sucanat or dehydrated cane juice
1 t baking powder
1/4 t baking soda
1/2 t salt
1 stick melted butter
1/4 cup buttermilk
2 eggs
1 t vanilla
2 cups frozen mixed berries
1/4 cup honey
2 T orange juice
2 T lemon juice

Combine the dry ingredients and set aside. In a medium bowl, beat the butter with the sugar. Add eggs and vanilla. Stir in the dry ingredients and milk. When well combined, fold in the berries. Bake at 350 degrees in a loaf pan for an hour or until golden brown. Remove from pan and allow to cool. Heat the honey and stir in the juices. Pour glaze evenly over the loaf. Serve warm.

Wild Rice

Native to North America, this grain is a powerhouse of nutrients. Wild rice contains more protein, minerals and B vitamins than wheat, barley and oats. The dark grains add an exotic look and deep flavor to many dishes, although they are most commonly used as a seasoning agent or garnishment for other rice dishes. This is partly due to the high cost of the grain, which is a result of somewhat primitive harvesting methods. While we often grumble about the modernizing of growing and harvesting methods, wild rice has not changed much in decades. The rice is still harvested by hand. Harvesters travel by canoe to the plants to gather the rice, which is then sent to the packaging plant.

Cooking times vary, but on average, 1 cup of wild rice will cook in 2 cups of water for an hour. It is ready when the grains burst open and the liquid is absorbed.

I love the nutty taste of wild rice and the dark color it imparts to the meal. My children, however, prefer it mellowed with plain rice for visual appeal and a milder flavor. Either way, it is a perfect side for many dishes and can adapt to just about any garnish. Try this elegant pomegranate pilaf for a special treat.

Pomegranate Wild Rice Pilaf

1/2 cup wild rice
1/2 cup brown rice
2 cups chicken stock
1 T coconut oil
1/4 cup chopped pecans
1 cup pomegranate seeds
1 scallion, chopped
1 T lemon zest
1 T parsley

Heat the oil over medium heat. Add the rice and stir to coat. Add the chicken stock and 1 cup water. Bring to a boil, cover and simmer for 40-60 minutes, until the liquid is absorbed. (Alternatively, cook rice in a rice cooker.) Stir in the lemon, seeds, nuts and herbs. Serve immediately.

Wine

Wine is an alcoholic beverage that has been consumed for millennia. Wine is typically made by fermenting grapes, but alcoholic beverages can be made by fermenting many foods. The drink has been common in just about every historic society, including ancient Greece and Rome. It is especially common among those who consume traditional Mediterranean diets, where it is consumed with meals.

The most popular wines are red, white and sparkling, which contain 10-14% alcohol. Many of the health benefits, however, can only be found in red wines.

The primary health benefit from wine is its function as a cardiotonic. This is found in moderate drinking, which can be defined as 1 glass a day for women and 1-2 glasses a day for men. Ideally, wine should be taken with meals to offset the alcohol content.

Both red and white wines have antibacterial compounds, which are especially effective against *Streptococcus.* This explains the traditional use of wine as an effective wound treatment.

Wine can be used in many recipes, especially those featuring meats. However, its primary role in the diet is to be consumed as-is.

Winter Squash

Winter squash is extremely nutrient dense. A one cup serving provides over 140% of the RDA for vitamin A. These mildly sweet yet savory vegetables also contain potassium, fiber, manganese, folate, copper, tryptophan, omega 3 acids, and vitamins C and B complex.

Squash are grown around the world, but they are native to South America. The winter varieties include butternut, acorn, hubbard, turban and pumpkins. While these varieties all vary greatly in size and color, they all share the same benefit of an abnormally long shelf life.

Winter squash varieties all offer plenty of phytonutrients. They also help to reduce symptoms of BPH, (benign prostatic hypertrophy) according to recent trials.

While squash adds a sweet taste and creamy texture to the meal, they do require some preparation. A quick slicing and baking is all that is usually needed to transform the thick food into a culinary treat.

Butternut Squash with Rosemary

1 stick butter
1 T rosemary
1 large butternut squash (can sub another large squash)

Peel the squash and cut into cubes. Bake at 375 degrees in a medium pan for 10 minutes. Set aside. In a large saucepan, melt the butter. When it is melted, add the rosemary and continue to cook until the butter is browned, about 1-2 minutes. Add the squash and stir while cooking until the butter is absorbed and the squash is tender, about 3-4 minutes. Serve warm.

Zucchini

Zucchini is a summer squash. While summer and winter squash have similar nutritional profiles, summer squash have several additional nutrients. Iron, vitamin K and zinc can be found in greater abundance in zucchini, though the exact differences among summer and winter squash will vary according to the growing conditions and type of squash.

Summer squash generally have shorter shelf lives than winter squash, so they need to be consumed quickly after purchasing, while winter squash can wait a few weeks. When preparing squash, summer squash have edible skin, so there is no need for peeling. Winter squash should be peeled or served in such a way that the peel can be easily avoided.

Zucchini Bites

2 medium zucchini
1 egg
1 T coconut oil
1/2 cup white wheat flour
2 chopped scallions
1 T parsley
2 T crumbled feta

Coarsely grate the zucchini, then place on towels to release some of the moisture. While the zucchini is sitting, whisk the egg with the oil, flour, herbs and cheese. Stir in the zucchini. Add salt and pepper to taste. Scoop by the teaspoonful onto a baking sheet. Bake at 375 degrees for 45 minutes or until brown and firm.

Resources:

Appendix One: Common Food Additives

It is important to note that not all chemicals present in food are considered food additives. Many are not even included on the label but are used in various stages of processing. A classic example of this would be pesticide use. While residue is present in food products, as evidenced by numerous studies and trials, the actual pesticides used through the various stages of production are not identified on the label. Other examples include antibiotics, fungicides, detergents, cleaning agents, hormones, drugs given to animals, solvents used to extract oils, pollutants found in the water or air, bleaching agents, and other environmental toxins that contaminate foods during the growth, processing or food preparation process. They can even include the chemical changes that occur during the processing process such as when high heat alters the molecular structure of an oil. These are technically known as indirect additives.

The only additives that are found on the label are intentional additives, those that are purposefully added to the ingredient list to serve a specific function such as food preservation, emulsification, flavor enhancing and other similar properties. Many of these are considered to be safe when consumed in moderate amounts, while others are linked with common health concerns. Most have been studied for short term consumption only; the safety of long term use is often unknown.

Likewise, most additives have been studied for limited consumption and many are even approved for limited use, but when the additive is found in 5-10 items in the diet daily, consumption often exceeds approved levels.

Below is a list of additives that are commonly found in foods. Many are quite safe, while the intake of others may need to be limited.

Acacia: see Gum Arabic

Aluminum (alum): Aluminum salts are found in food products under various names, but typically the alum- prefix identifies the ingredient. While aluminum is a naturally occurring material, its abundant use in food products, cosmetic products and cookware has brought its safety into question. In particular, it has been linked with dementia, and other cognitive disorders. Sodium aluminum phosphate is found in many baking powders, and foil and cookware are also contributing sources of the material. Given the potential health concerns and lack of information regarding long term use at such high levels, it is generally considered ideal to avoid aluminum where possible.

Annatto: Annatto is a natural coloring agent that is also a natural spice. It can be used for naturally dyed eggs and naturally colored foods. As a natural supplement, it carries a great safety record and is primarily found in yellowish foods such as dairy products and cake mixes.

Artificial Flavor: This is a catch all term that covers many additives and indirect additives. Research has linked many artificial flavors with adverse behavior in children and reduced attention capabilities. As an artificial food, artificial flavors do not play a role in the real foods diet.

Aspartame (AminoSweet, Nutrasweet, Equal): Aspartame, though rebranded as a natural sweetener, amino sweet, is anything but healthy. Though it has a long standing use in food products and has become the most common artificial sweetener, found in nearly 6,000 food products, its safety is questionable at best. Many studies have linked the product with migraines, worsening of seizures and even increased risk of brain tumors in animals. Its breakdown includes phenylalanine, so anyone with PKU should avoid it. Like all artificial sweeteners, the questionable safety can be avoided by using natural sugars in a balanced diet.

BHA, BHT (butylated hydroxyanisole and butylated hydroxytolune): These petroleum byproducts are used in food preservation where they serve as preservatives, extending the shelf life of various products. Initially developed for non-food items, the vast majority of current BHA and BHT is still for non food sources. It is used in many dry goods, seasonings and processed "instant" foods. Safety concerns, such as potential carcinogenic effects, documented ability to disrupt metabolic intercellular processes and liver toxicity have caused the FDA to issue limits on allowable levels in foods. There is also concern that, when metabolized, the products convert to stronger carcinogens within the body. In England, BHT is prohibited, but many other countries still allow it. Considering the lack of safety assurance from the researchers, healthy diets would benefit from the avoidance of such questionable preservatives.

Calcium Chloride, Carbonate, Citrate: These are known as calcium salts, and are sources of the valuable mineral, calcium. While often found as an additive in many food products, they are also used widely in supplements. Their usefulness in food products is not necessarily with your health as the goal; calcium salts help to emulsify various foods and as dough conditioners. They also help to balance the acidity of various foods and supplements. While they may not be the best bioavailable source of calcium, their intake is not worrisome.

Caramel Color: While many assume that caramel color is an extract from the syrupy treat that adorns ice cream desserts, it is actually an entirely synthetic additive more properly identified as an artificial color. Caramel color is most commonly found in carbonated beverages, but various foods and snacks contain the additive. In animal studies, caramel coloring has decreased immune function and affected the thymus gland. Most foods that contain caramel coloring are highly processed and are not included in a real foods diet.

Citric Acid: This additive can be extracted from citrus fruits, but is more commonly obtained from whey. New production methods utilize fungal compounds, so those on antifungal diets may wish to restrict intake. It can be found in many foods, typically serving as a flavor enhancer or acidic compound to enhance preservatives. Naturally occurring in many foods, citric acid is quite safe and despite modern production techniques could still be considered natural.

Corn Syrup: Corn syrup and high fructose corn syrup are the controversial sweeteners obtained from corn. Corn is a subsidized crop, making it artificially inexpensive, thus an ideal food ingredient for low quality food products. It is found in many foods, but has been linked to numerous health concerns, including obesity, diabetes, cardiac concerns and other modern epidemics. Additionally, corn syrup typically comes from non-organic GMO corn, which increases the amount of indirect additives, the long term effects of which are unknown.

EDTA / Calcium Disodium EDTA: Calcium disodium EDTA is used medicinally as a chelator. Chelate literally means "claw" and a chelator is used to bind (and eventually remove) heavy metals from the body. In foods, it is used to preserve various products, usually condiments of some sort. This prevents metals from changing the color or flavor of the food, but many are concerned that it may deplete our own stores of zinc and copper due to its ability to bind to them. While currently approved for food use, its safety is questionable. It has been found to be cytotoxic in animals and is thought to cause reproductive and developmental effects. Due to its widespread use, it has become classified as a persistent organic pollutant.

Glycerides (monoglycerides, diglycerides): These are naturally occurring fats that are used in food products as thickeners and emulsifiers in items such as condiments, butter substitutes and dairy products. While they are naturally occurring, many food additives are chemically synthesized so it is important to be aware of which type of glyceride is in the product.

Glycerin: Glycerin is used in herbal medicine as a menstruum - an agent that serves as the extracting liquid for the active compounds - and a preserving agent. It can be found in food items as a thickener. It can be naturally occurring and slightly sweet, and it is a natural humectant, which means it attracts water. It is also used externally in cosmetics as an emollient in soaps, lotions and other skin care products. As a preferred primary ingredient in natural medicines, it has a long standing history of safety.

Guar Gum: This naturally occurring compound is extracted from the guar plant. It serves as a thickener and binds foods together. It can be found in many brands of ice cream, processed cheeses and condiments. There is some concern about consumption by pregnant women, but for the general public, it is considered to be quite safe. It is even used as a supplement for various health purposes.

Gum Arabic: Gum Arabic helps to keep mixtures combined and serves as a thickener. It is most commonly found in glazes, sauces, jelly-type candies and fruit spreads. It can also be found in chewing gum, beer and carbonated beverages. The gum comes from the acacia tree, native to Africa, and has actually been used for over a thousand years. It does not pose substantial safety concerns, but is highly allergenic. Unfortunately it is typically used in processed foods, so its safety is not usually the concern with its consumption.

Hydrolyzed Vegetable Protein (HVP): This additive can be produced using petroleum distillates, leaving residues that are concerning, and the hydrolytic process is questionable among health professionals. It involves using an agent to split proteins into individual amino acids, resulting in free glutamate. Many believe this combines with sodium creating MSG. Regardless, it is certainly not a real food, and the use of HVP in soups, sauces and even baby food is one that is best avoided.

Lecithin (soy lecithin): Lecithin is naturally occurring in eggs and can be purchased as a natural health supplement. In foods, however, most lecithin is obtained from soy or, to a lesser extent, corn. It is an emulsifier and as a natural health supplement is taken to help cholesterol levels, particularly triglycerides. However, soy lecithin used in most food products is not the same thing that naturally occurs in eggs. It is a byproduct of soybean oil production, extracted using various solvents. For those sensitive or allergic to soy products, the claim has been made that soy lecithin is free of soy, but many claim to still experience negative results. While natural and organic lecithin can serve as a healthy supplement, most soy lecithin found in foods could not be classified as a real food or real food extract.

Modified Food Starch: A modified food starch, as the name suggests, is a starch (carbohydrate) that has been modified to change certain characteristics such as its ability to dissolve or its texture. In processed foods, they are used as thickeners but they can also be found as anti-caking agents in packaged mixes. While they are considered to be safe food additives, many have questioned that safety and linked the substance with MSG formation and digestion problems. Nonetheless, the modification and processing of starches is not found on a diet of real foods and generally offers no nutritional benefit.

Monosodium Glutamate (MSG): MSG is a controversial additive that is based on naturally occurring compounds, confusing many about its origins and safety. While many are familiar with the 4 tastes: sweet, salty, sour and bitter, few know about the fifth: umami. Umami, sometimes referred to as *savory,* is the taste experience that occurs when rich foods such as red wine, hard cheeses or long simmering red sauces are ingested. The comforting savory taste of such foods is generally the result of long hours dedicated by someone with vast experience in the art of food and drink production. Once this was discovered, shortcuts were sought and the combination of glutamic acid with sodium, when combined with food, appears to trick the body into tasting the umami sensation. While many would argue that the two are chemically similar, thus both safe, many experts disagree, classifying MSG as a neurotoxin, contributing to headaches, numbness, chest pains, and tingling. More serious cases include neurological disorders such as dystonia. Many of these symptoms are commonly called "Chinese restaurant syndrome" but the reality is that most restaurant food contains MSG, as it is a common ingredient in various sauces, including pizza sauce, hot wing sauce, many Asian inspired sauces as well as Italian sauces and numerous other items, even the macaroni and cheese so commonly found in children's menus.

Nitrates: Nitrates are used in the process of curing meats such as ham, bacon, hot dogs and sausage. While they help the meat retain its color, many would argue that color retention is far less of a problem than the health concerns relates to the use of nitrates and nitrites (see below). When combined with amines in digestive juices, nitrates form potent carcinogens known as nitrosamines. Obviously such substances don't have a place in a real foods diet. (It is important to note that the phrase "no nitrates added" is often valuable as minimal amounts of nitrates are naturally occurring in various vegetables. These amounts are extremely low, but explain the use of the term "added" to the meat product.)

Nitrites: Nitrites are the more stable relative of nitrates. They are used to retain colors in meats during the curing process, just like nitrates. They also protect against the growth of harmful bacteria in meat products. However, like nitrates, when they interact with amines either in the digestive process or in the food product, to form nitrosamines. Nitrates also have the ability to form other carcinogens, amyl and butyl nitrites. Like nitrates, a real foods diet would not contain such potentially harmful substances. Processed meats, if desired, can be found in health foods stores that have been cured without nitrates or nitrites.

Parabens: Parabens are often associated with cosmetic products, where they have earned a negative reputation, but many foods and pharmaceuticals contain them as well. Their main function is to preserve foods and medicines. However, if I don't want to apply lotions with parabens to my skin, I certainly don't want to intentionally ingest anything containing parabens.

Pectin: This naturally occurring compound can be found in many fruits and helps them form the gel like texture we enjoy in jams and preserves. It also serves as a binding agent and / or thickener in other food products. They are safe and even have medicinal uses for the treatment of diarrhea.

Polysorbate 60: This is made from sorbitol and serves as an emulsifier in many food products. Many processed foods contain polysorbate 60 and thought it has been initially considered to be safe, further study has been recommended by many experts because the effects of some of the compounds used in its production are unknown.

Propolyne Glycol: This is made from a byproduct of petroleum refining, propylene gas. It is used in food production to blend foods together and as a solvent. It can be found in various foods including beverages, pastries, ice cream, chocolate, baked goods and condiments. Propolyne glycol is also found in many cosmetics, where is serves as an emulsifier and penetration enhancer. Externally, safety concerns regarding potential links to fertility and cancer risks have been raised by environmental health organizations and endocrine disrupting potential is a concern with high doses. Internally, it is considered to be safe by many authorities, however, in Europe, its allowable food uses are extremely limited.

Rennet: This is an enzyme, obtained from the intestines of cows, which induces the curdling of milk that results in cheese. It is found in cheese products and is safe for consumption. However, those that prefer to avoid such products can also obtain cheese made with vegetable based rennet.

Saccharin: This sweetener has seen its share of controversy. After initial approval, the FDA suggested a ban on the product, which was met with resistance by the public, resulting in its current availability. The EPA considers it to be a potential carcinogen, and many health experts agree, as the substance may be particularly harmful for pregnant women and children. Nonetheless, it is still available in many diet foods as a sugar substitute.

Silicates (silicon dioxide): Not to be confused with salicylates, silicates are salts from silica oxides. In food products they are found in baking ingredients and mixes. While silica, an important substance for the human body, is related to silicon, the agents used in food preparation do not appear to provide any nutritional benefit, and the bioavailability of the substance is unknown. Studies don't seem to support one side or another, but without answers to questions of safety, it is hard to comfortably consume the substance.

Sodium Benzoate: Also known as benzoic acid, sodium benzoate is primarily used in food products as a preservative or flavoring enhancer. It can be found most often in candies and processed foods such as margarine and assorted condiments. When consumed, it is metabolized by the liver. It has a long history of use in the food industry and is naturally occurring in many whole foods and herbs. While it can be allergenic and does put a mild strain on the liver, it is one of the safest food preservatives used in conventional foods, when ingested in small amounts. Food preservatives in general, however, can be avoided by preparing meals at home, using fresh natural ingredients.

Sodium Bicarbonate: also known as baking soda

Sodium Chloride: also known as table salt

Sorbitol: This can be a naturally occurring sugar, but is also produced by chemically modifying corn sugar. In food products, it serves many purposes including controlling texture and crystallization. The body does not metabolize it as a sugar and it is assumed to be safe, but more research is necessary to ensure that increased amounts of a modified product are actually safe.

Soy Lecithin: see Lecithin

Soy Protein Isolate (TVP): When soybean oil is extracted from the plant, the leftover residue is processed to make soy protein isolate. This substance is sold individually as a vegetarian protein option, but is also included in many milk substitutes, particularly baby formula, and is available in many seasonings, flavorings and condiments. While small amounts may be safe, this is not a complete protein substitute and the processing means that it is not a whole, real food.

Sucralose: Sucralose is a newer sugar substitute, produced by alternating three chemical groups in sugar with chlorine. As a newer substitute, research on safety, particularly long term safety is limited, and as an artificially processed food, it is not a part of a real foods diet.

Sucrose: also known as sugar

Sulfites: These are preservatives used to prevent microbial contamination of many foods and drinks. They are generally recognized as safe, but there is concern that they can increase the actions of carcinogens. While they are not carcinogenic themselves, this behavior would be troublesome if it is the case. They are also known to cause reactions in sensitive individuals, causing diarrhea, nausea, headaches, and worsening of asthmatic symptoms.

TBHQ: Tertiary butylhydroquinone is a butane gas derivative of petroleum and is quite new to the food industry. It serves as a preservative and is toxic in even moderate amounts if ingested. More specifically, it is a neurotoxin and alters red blood cell activity, which can lead to numerous health and behavioral concerns. While allowable food usage is restricted, this substance is not a part of a real foods diet in any amount.

Turmeric: This frightening sounding additive is actually an herb in the ginger family, used in food products as a natural yellow coloring agent. Turmeric provides anti-inflammatory properties and has been researched (with promising results) as a potential treatment for cancer and IBS. It is rich in antioxidants and supplementation often results in improved liver function and lowered cholesterol.

TVP: see Soy Protein Isolate

Xanthan Gum: This is a thickening agent produced when bacteria is introduced to corn sugar. The two interact, forming a thick sludge, which when dried, acts like corn starch or guar gum in food items. As a corn product, it is somewhat controversial, particularly considering the quality of corn sugar likely used in its production. In food products, it is most commonly found in gluten free items, as it acts as a substitute for gluten. While nothing can replace the actions of gluten, it does help lighten many gluten free baked goods. It is also used medicinally as a laxative.

Yeast: Yeast typically refers to baker's yeast, which is controversial in a real foods diet. While baker's yeast may appear to be a real food, it is actually a specific strand of yeast bred to speed and regulate the baking process. Research has shown that foods prepared with naturally occurring yeasts (fermentation) do not deplete the body of iron, magnesium and zinc like those with baker's yeast can, and they contribute to better gluten toleration by reducing the gluten content of the baked good. While baker's yeast may not be a bad food, it is not the ideal option.

Appendix Two: Sweetening Options

Most cookbooks call for some amount of white sugar in every recipe. Making substitutions can often be tricky, especially when liquid sweeteners are used. Details on making such substitutions are included with each sweetener description, but trial and error is often the best method of modifying a favorite recipe.

Agave Nectar: Agave nectar has a glycemic index of 11, making it a great substitute when used in moderation. It contains fructose rather than glucose, which places a greater burden on the liver, but the fructose is not concentrated as it is in HFCS. Nonetheless, I do not recommend using agave nectar as a full time substitute, but it is a healthy option for occasional use or when combined with other sweeteners.

Artificial Sweeteners: These are chemicals that offer the sweetness of sugar without the calories. While popular with habitual dieters and those that produce "diet" foods, these are never a whole food, and may cause harm to our bodies. The FDA currently approves only 5 as sugar substitutes, and the FDA felt the need to establish an ADI (accepted daily intake) for each of the 5. The ADI ranges from 5-50 mg per day, depending on the sweetener.

Brown Rice Syrup: This sweetener is thick and syrupy, just like corn syrup. It is flavorless and works perfectly in all recipes that call for corn syrup - particularly those that just don't work well with other substitutions. Organic is a must.

Dehydrated Cane Juice: Dehydrated cane juice is a middle ground between white sugar and an evaporated cane sugar such as sucanat or rapadura. The refining process is similar to both, leaving in some of the natural minerals but crystallizing the sugar and stripping other minerals. In our home, we use it sparingly when no other sugar substitute will work. It has the taste and texture of white sugar, but a light brown appearance.

Fructose: Fructose has the same chemical formula as glucose but a different molecular structure. It comes from fruit, and is generally marketed to diabetics. Fructose has no vitamins, minerals or enzymes, so it is essentially no better than white sugar (glucose). It does not spike the blood sugar as dramatically as white sugar, but it is a processed food, far from its natural or whole state. It is metabolized by the liver, which makes it a trade off in terms of damage.

Honey: Honey is 25% sweeter than white sugar and contains vitamins and minerals. It also contains healthy antioxidants. It is actually a combination of sugars, so it can give a quick release of glucose into the blood as well as a slow release. This, combined with the provided nutrients, makes honey a good substitute over traditional sugar. Honey has a general glycemic index much lower than white sugar. It is important to remember though, that honey still raises the blood sugar and should be consumed in moderation. When substituting for sugar, use 3/4 cup to 1 cup sugar and reduce the liquids by about 3 T for each cup of sugar that was removed.

Maple Syrup: Maple syrup is a natural sweetener made from the sap of maple trees. While it contains many vitamins and minerals, it does still have a fairly high glycemic index and the potential to raise blood sugar. It is much sweeter than sugar so, like honey, only a fraction can sweeten just as well.

Molasses: Molasses is the thick by product of sugar production. Blackstrap molasses comes from the third process, meaning it contains the greatest source of nutrients that were stripped from the table sugar.

In the case of non organic sugar, it also will contain the greatest concentration of contaminants, including pesticides. For this reason, I always suggest organic molasses. It is a mineral rich sweetener with a strong flavor, ideal for gingerbread or other strong foods.

Turbinado Sugar (or raw sugar): This is basically regular white sugar with a little of the molasses added back in to give it a more natural or raw look. It is no better than white sugar and still spikes the blood sugar, robs the body of minerals and is not a whole food.

Stevia: This herb is 300 times as sweet as sugar. It is also reputed to prevent tooth decay and cavities. It can be found in the herbal section of a health food store, usually as a glycerite. It is best used in drinks such as lemonade and sweet tea. (Stevia has a zero glycemic index.)

Sucanat: (SUgar CAne NATural; also sold under the name Rapadura): Sucanat is literally ground sugar cane. It has a granular texture (resembling dirt) that is still full of all the naturally occurring vitamins and minerals. Sucanat contains potassium, vitamins A, B1, B2 and B6, calcium, iron, magnesium, zinc, copper, chromium and phosphorus. The chromium is noteworthy since chromium is commonly taken to balance blood sugar. This may be why sucanat has a naturally low glycemic index. Since the molasses has not been removed from the cane, sucanat has a rich, natural flavor that enhances most foods. Sucanat or rapadura can still spike blood sugar if eaten in excess, but moderate amounts offer a pretty balanced glycemic load.

Xylitol: Xylitol is a five-carbon sugar alcohol that is used as a sugar substitute. It is as sweet as glucose, but with only 2/3 the calories. It is typically made from corn and promoted as a healthy sugar for the teeth. It can be harmful to dogs and other household pets, so use caution when pets are around.

Appendix Three: Naturally Leavened Bread

As covered in the Seven Confusing Foods chapter, modern bread, even homemade whole wheat bread, is still not technically a traditional, real food. Using natural sourdough starters to ferment the dough with various strands of yeast and useful bacteria helps to reduce the gluten content, decrease the glycemic load and increase the bioavailability of magnesium, zinc and iron. These are important health benefits for all of us!

Naturally leavened breads are often considered to be quite overwhelming, but the technique is quite simple after a little experience is obtained. Sourdough starters (often called *mother*) can be purchased online or "caught" from the air, but should never contain any baker's yeast. The Vintage Remedies Network is a great source of regional tips and recipes from other like minded individuals. I've also included some of my personal favorites below:

Whole Wheat Loaf

1 cup active sourdough "mother"
5 cups whole wheat flour
2 cups water
1 T honey

2 t salt
2 T oil

Mix the mother culture with 1 cup flour. Combine well. Add another cup of flour and half the water. Leave for 4 hours at room temperature. Add the rest of the ingredients. Knead until the dough is a smooth ball. You can add up to another half a cup of water as needed for a soft, yet firm dough.

Form into 2 loaves and place in baking pans. To form the loaves, roll each half into a rectangle. Fold up into thirds like a letter. Gently flatten again and roll up tightly. Place into a greased pan seam side down. Let rise until doubled, which will take 2-3 hours at room temperature. I like to do this final rise in the oven with the light on. It will rise faster, however, so keep an eye on it. I also cover the dough with a warm, damp towel. This keeps it from drying out.

Gently score the middle of the bread. Bake at 400 degrees for 30-40 minutes. Do not open the oven for the first 30 minutes. The bread is ready when it is golden brown and begins to slightly pull away form the pan.

You don't have to have a starter that is trained exclusively on whole wheat to make this bread, but it does help. For picky eaters, substitute 1/2 the wheat flour for white. Or, try white wheat flour. It is still a whole wheat flour, but ground from white wheat instead of red, which gives it a lighter flavor.

Variations:

Add any of the following to the final stage:
1 T Italian herbs
1/2 cup cranberries and 1/2 cup walnuts
1/2 cup raisins and 1/2 cup pecans
1 T cinnamon and 1/2 cup raisins or currants
1/4 cup sun dried tomatoes and 1 t basil
1/4 cup grated cheddar cheese and 1 t garlic puree

Herbed Dinner Rolls

For herbed dinner rolls, follow the bread dough recipe. Add the Italian herbs to the dough at the end. Instead of forming into loaves, divide into 12 or 36 small balls. Dip each into melted butter and place into muffin tins. (If using 36 balls, place 3 to a tin for a cloverleaf roll.) Let rise until doubled. Bake at 375 for 25-35 minutes. To pre-bake, bake for 15 minutes, then remove from the pan and freeze. When you are ready to prepare them, remove from the freezer and place on a cookie sheet. Bake at 350 for 15-20 minutes or until golden brown.

Pizza Dough

Pizza dough is dramatically improved by naturally leavened dough. The tangy taste of a sourdough is enhanced by the rich flavors of the sauce and toppings.

1 cup active sourdough "mother"
2.5 cups whole wheat flour
2 cups white flour
2 cups water
2 t salt
2 t olive oil
optional: 1 t basil or Italian seasoning for flavored crust

Combine all of the ingredients in a large stand mixer or large bowl, stirring by hand. Knead until the dough forms a smooth ball. Add up to another 1/4 cup water, if needed.

Place the dough in a greased bowl to rest 60-90 minutes. It is ready when it has doubled in size. Divide into 4 rounds and let rest 15 minutes. Flatten out into rounds. Top with desired toppings. (To prevent soggy crust, brush with olive oil prior to adding the sauce.) Bake at 500 degrees for 8-10 minutes.

Holiday Rolls

If they fall asleep with visions of sugarplums, they should wake with the scent of sweet cinnamon breakfast rolls. These typically naughty treats are made much healthier in this recipe.

Follow the recipe for whole wheat bread, but use half wheat and half white flour. Add another 2 T honey to the dough and substitute 1/2 cup milk for part of the water. When it is ready to form into a loaf for the pan, roll out into 2 large rectangles. Spread softened butter over the top of each. Mix together 1/2 cup pecans, 1/2 cup raisins or currants, 1/2 cup sucanat and 1 T cinnamon (for each rectangle). Sprinkle over the butter and spread evenly. Begin with one end and roll up into a log. Slice into 3/4 inch rounds and place in a greased baking sheet.

Let rise in the fridge overnight. Remove from the cold and place at room temperature for one to three hours or until the rolls are fluffy. (This time frame will depend on the heat of your kitchen.) Place in a 350 degree oven and bake for an hour. Serve hot.

Pancakes

Even pancakes can be improved upon with a natural dough starter. My favorite part about these pancakes is that they are the only pancakes I have seen that are not laden with milk! The tangy flavor goes well with a sweet maple syrup or molasses. For fruity pancakes, toss a handful of berries onto the top after pouring into the pan.

1 cup active sourdough "mother"
1 cup water
1 cup wheat flour
1/2 cup buttermilk
dash salt
2 T butter
1 egg

Mix together the mother culture, water and flour. Let rest overnight in the fridge. Remove from the fridge and add the rest of the ingredients. Melt butter on the griddle over medium high heat. Scoop 1/4 cup at a time over hot butter. Cook 3-4 minutes on each side. Serve hot with butter and maple syrup.

For Further Learning

Real foods, traditional medicine and natural wellness are important considerations for modern families concerned with the status of the current food system, the healthcare situation and / or the sustainability of common lifestyles. Yet, few of use were taught these natural living techniques during childhood, and even those that were can benefit from continuing education through modern advancements in the field of natural health.

The Vintage Remedies School of Natural Health (www.VintageRemedies.com) was founded by Jessie Hawkins in the summer of 2007 to meet the growing demand for a different kind of wellness education. Since that time, it has become a unique offering in the ever growing field of natural health. Offering distance learning opportunities, multiple programs with a solid base in modern evidence based integrative medicine, yet founded on biblically sound principles, and backed by a dependable, reputable name in natural health allows us to stand apart from the growing number of educational opportunities available today.

Our resources include not only wellness educational programs, but also continuing education for both healthcare professionals in need of CEUs and for wellness students and graduates desiring to stay on top of the current research. We also provide workshops and conferences throughout the country as well as virtual events available through our online classroom to cover various topics.

All of our distance learning programs are completely self paced and can be started and completed on your own schedule. We offer online resources for networking with other students and personal assistance and feedback from our office to evaluate your progress and identify areas in need of additional work, in addition to the regular grading process for unit work. Furthermore, each of our programs were designed to integrate fully with the other courses we offer. Upon completion of one course, many students choose to continue their education with another of our programs . When this happens, many of the credits transfer directly to the new program and the cost is adjusted to reflect any coursework previously completed in a previous program with us.

Each course includes the Vintage Remedies textbook(s), a copy of *The Handbook of Vintage Remedies*, an herbal medicine making kit, admission to the student only message boards, evaluation and feedback from our staff as well as personal "one on one" time with Jessie and discounted admission to all Vintage Remedies events.

Our distance learning programs include a **Natural Wellness** course, providing 120 hours of study over approximately 4 -5 months. This is our introductory program for those new to the subject. Each of the 8 units are taken from our advanced program and if the student decides to continue with another program upon completion, 100% of the cost can be applied towards another course and the grades will be transferred as well.

More advanced programs include the **Family Herbalist Course**, the **Clinical Master Herbalist Course**, and the **Holistic Wellness Professional Program**.

Our Family Herbalist program is one of the most comprehensive and thorough family herbalist programs available. This "Herbology 101" course takes a whole person, integrative approach to the modern health concerns the average family is likely to face, matching them with evidence based and time tested ancient medicine. Featuring prevention, herbal preparations, aromatherapy, and a lengthy materia medica, our Family Herbalist program teaches students how to care for their families using reliable and effective natural medicine from a Biblical perspective. It also serves to prepare the serious student for one of our advanced programs suitable for a clinical practice or professional career.

This intensive program is divided into 26 topical units and provides 360 study hours to the learner. It can be finished in a year by completing one unit each two weeks.

Sample unit topics for the Family Herbalist course include:

- Holistic Nutrition
- Prevention in Childbearing
- Vaccinations
- Modern Childhood Epidemics
- Pharmacognosy and Herbal Medicine
- Materia Medica - over 100 herbs!
- Herbal Preparations
- Aromatherapy
- Prevention in Homekeeping

The Vintage Remedies Clinical Master Herbalist program prepares aspiring herbalists to enter the field of herbalism fully equipped with the training and experience necessary for success. By combining the art and science of natural medicine, our clinical Master Herbalists learn how to observe, distinguish and prevent susceptibilities and patterns of disease using a holistic model of care. This whole person, integrative approach is necessary to the understanding of effective herbal medicine.

This program is ideal for those desiring to pursue careers as clinical herbalists, for licensed medical practitioners ready to enter the field of integrative medicine, and for individuals aspiring to become a recognized professionals in the field of herbal medicine. Our study topics also include kinesiology, environmental health, traditional diets, biblical herbs, epidemiology, recognition and reversal of nutritional deficiencies, psychoneuroimmunology, and much more.

The program uses the Family Herbalist Course as an introduction and includes 42 additional units, covering all aspects of education necessary to become a competent herbalist. An emphasis is placed on relevant, current health concerns and up to date scientific evidence, placing our graduates at the cutting edge of the field! With a combined total of up to 1800 hours, our program is one of the most thorough and comprehensive available. Sample unit topics for the Clinical Master Herbalist course include:

- History and Philosophy of Herbal Medicine
- Evidence Based Medicine
- Phytochemistry

- General Pharmacology
- Advanced Aromatherapy
- Toxicity, Reactions, Interactions and Contraindications
- Adaptogens
- Environmental Health
- Epidemiology
- Psychoneuroimmunology
- Advanced Nutrition
- Intake Strategies
- Gestation and Lactation

Finally, the Holistic Wellness Professional program covers every aspect of natural health imaginable! In addition to herbalism, this unique new program includes homeopathy, enzymatic therapy, reflexology, flower remedies, aromatherapy, naturopathy, nutrition and sustainable living. With a focus on prevention and healthy lifestyles, our Holistic Wellness Professional course provides the training to accurately promote healthy and balanced living within your home and community. Like all of our courses, this program teaches reliable and effective natural medicine from a Biblical perspective.

This comprehensive program is divided into 44 units, covering a variety of aspects within natural health and provides a total of 960 hours of study. Sample unit topics from the Holistic Wellness Professional Program include:

- Food or Medicine: Ancient Dietary Practices
- Psychoneuroimmunology
- Enzymatic Therapies
- Weight Management
- Pathophysiology
- Detoxification, Antioxidants and Phytonutrients
- Integrative Medicine for Women's Health
- Environmental Health
- Sustainable Living
- Epidemiology and Statistics
- Homeopathy
- Naturopathy
- Lifestyle Consulting
- Natural Preparations

Index:

Recipe Index:

About The Author

Jessie Hawkins, founded Vintage Remedies to answer the growing need of women and mothers everywhere to have a reliable source to turn to for answers to their natural health questions. What began as a small consulting practice blossomed into multiple written works, an extensive website filled with tips and formulas for natural living and more recently, the Vintage Remedies School of Natural Health, which educates individuals throughout the world about the safe and effective use of herbal remedies and natural health.

When she is not consulting, writing or speaking, Jessie stays busy maintaining her family vegetable and herb gardens, exploring new ideas in the kitchen with her family and traveling with her husband to various new places. She lives in a Nashville suburb with her husband Matthew and their four children.

Other Works by Jessie:

The Handbook of Vintage Remedies, 2009, 2012
The Vintage Remedies Guide to Bread, 20012

Find Jessie at:

www.JessieHawkins.com
www.VintageRemedies.com